Breast Elastography
Basic Principles and Interpretation of Clinical Cases

Breast Elastography
Basic Principles and Interpretation of Clinical Cases

Christina An. Gkali MD candidate PhD
Resident
Department of Radiology
"Alexandra" General Hospital of Athens
Athens, Greece

Constantine Dimitrakakis MD PhD
Associate Professor
Department of Obstetrics and Gynecology
Medical School, University of Athens
Athens, Greece
Head, Department of Breast Surgery
"Alexandra" General Hospital of Athens
Athens, Greece

Maria Sotiropoulou MD PhD
Senior Consultant/Director
Department of Histopathology
"Alexandra" General Hospital of Athens
Athens, Greece

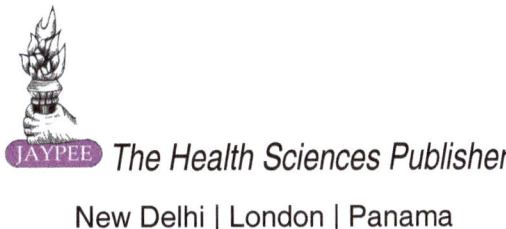

JAYPEE *The Health Sciences Publisher*

New Delhi | London | Panama

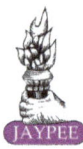

Jaypee Brothers Medical Publishers (P) Ltd

Headquarters
Jaypee Brothers Medical Publishers (P) Ltd.
4838/24, Ansari Road, Daryaganj
New Delhi 110 002, India
Phone: +91-11-43574357
Fax: +91-11-43574314
E-mail: jaypee@jaypeebrothers.com

Overseas Offices

J.P. Medical Ltd.
83, Victoria Street, London
SW1H 0HW (UK)
Phone: +44-20 3170 8910
Fax: +44(0)20 3008 6180
E-mail: info@jpmedpub.com

Jaypee-Highlights Medical Publishers Inc.
City of Knowledge, Bld. 235, 2nd Floor, Clayton
Panama City, Panama
Phone: +1 507-301-0496
Fax: +1 507-301-0499
E-mail: cservice@jphmedical.com

Jaypee Brothers Medical Publishers (P) Ltd.
17/1-B, Babar Road, Block-B, Shaymali
Mohammadpur, Dhaka-1207
Bangladesh
Mobile: +08801912003485
E-mail: jaypeedhaka@gmail.com

Jaypee Brothers Medical Publishers (P) Ltd.
Bhotahity, Kathmandu, Nepal
Phone: +977-9741283608
E-mail: kathmandu@jaypeebrothers.com

Website: www.jaypeebrothers.com
Website: www.jaypeedigital.com

© 2018, Jaypee Brothers Medical Publishers

The views and opinions expressed in this book are solely those of the original contributor(s)/author(s) and do not necessarily represent those of editor(s) of the book.

All rights reserved. No part of this publication may be reproduced, stored or transmitted in any form or by any means, electronic, mechanical, photocopying, recording or otherwise, without the prior permission in writing of the publishers.

All brand names and product names used in this book are trade names, service marks, trademarks or registered trademarks of their respective owners. The publisher is not associated with any product or vendor mentioned in this book.

Medical knowledge and practice change constantly. This book is designed to provide accurate, authoritative information about the subject matter in question. However, readers are advised to check the most current information available on procedures included and check information from the manufacturer of each product to be administered, to verify the recommended dose, formula, method and duration of administration, adverse effects and contraindications. It is the responsibility of the practitioner to take all appropriate safety precautions. Neither the publisher nor the author(s)/editor(s) assume any liability for any injury and/or damage to persons or property arising from or related to use of material in this book.

This book is sold on the understanding that the publisher is not engaged in providing professional medical services. If such advice or services are required, the services of a competent medical professional should be sought.

Every effort has been made where necessary to contact holders of copyright to obtain permission to reproduce copyright material. If any have been inadvertently overlooked, the publisher will be pleased to make the necessary arrangements at the first opportunity. The **CD/DVD-ROM** (if any) provided in the sealed envelope with this book is complimentary and free of cost. **Not meant for sale.**

Inquiries for bulk sales may be solicited at: jaypee@jaypeebrothers.com

Breast Elastography: Basic Principles and Interpretation of Clinical Cases

First Edition: **2018**

ISBN: 978-93-5270-057-8

Printed at

Dedicated to

The memory of my father, and my husband Michael for his tolerance and endurance.

—**Christina An. Gkali**

Preface

Ultrasound imaging is a first-line imaging modality for a wide range of indications, playing a major role in screening, diagnosis, and therapeutic interventions for various diseases and pathologies. However, even with enormous improvements in recent years, conventional ultrasound is limited in its ability to differentiate between the mechanical properties of tissue, which can be important in assessing the morphology and physiology of focal or diffuse disease.

Ultrasound elastography was initially introduced as a new imaging method adjunct to ultrasound in order to overcome ultrasonography limitations, such as increased number of unnecessary biopsies.

The use of more than one imaging tools can provide overall higher diagnostic accuracy than one imaging modality alone. This proved true when adding elastography to conventional ultrasound and when using multiple elastography technologies in cooperation.

This book refers to medical professionals who wish to practice breast ultrasound elastography. The book aims to provide the specialist with a detailed practical guide to the techniques of breast elastography (provided by our equipment—Acuson Siemens, S2000) and the interpretation of images obtained. Also, the last part of the book presents some pitfalls of elastography.

It is hoped that the majority of those who practice breast elastography will find this book readily accessible and affordable and that they will come to regard it as an invaluable starter manual and practical handbook.

I hope, I have been able to communicate some of my passion and enthusiasm for breast ultrasound and by extension, ultrasound elastography and that by reading this book others will come to feel this for themselves.

Christina An. Gkali

Acknowledgments

I would like to thank Constantine Dimitrakakis and Maria Sotiropoulou who have contributed chapters. Thank them for their hard work, consistency and kind response to my request to be contributors of this book. Without their contribution the writing of this book would have been impossible.

In addition to the co-authors listed above, I would also like to thank the following for their willingness to provide helpful and constructive feedback and supply illustrations:

Monali Padwal, MD, Clinical Manager, G.I Application, Siemens Medical Solutions, USA, Inc.

Amy Wilkinson, BS, AMS, RDMS, RSMSK, Clinical Specialist Ultrasound, HC US PMCM CA, Siemens Medical Solutions, Ultrasound, USA.

Litsa Bouzika, MSc Medical Physics, Siemens Healthineers, Greece, and Helen Cleminson, Clinical Marketing Manager, General Imaging and Radiology, CMEA at Siemens Healthcare.

Special thanks to Athanasios Chalazonitis, MD, MPH, PhD, Head of Radiology Department, "Alexandra" General Hospital of Athens, Greece and Eleni Feida, MD, Head of Breast Radiology Department, "Alexandra" General Hospital of Athens, Greece, for their support.

Finally, I would like to thank Lia Angela Moulopoulos—Professor of Radiology, Aris Antoniou—Associate Professor of Radiology, and Elias Primetis—Lecturer, Faculty Member, from Aretaieio Hospital Medical School, University of Athens, Greece.

I would also like to thank Mr Jitendar P Vij (Group Chairman), Mr Ankit Vij (Group President), Ms Chetna Malhotra Vohra (Associate Director-Content Strategy), Ms Nedup Denka Bhutia (Development Editor), and the entire team of Jaypee Brothers Medical Publishers, New Delhi, India, for their outstanding efforts in bringing out this book in record time.

Christina An. Gkali

Contents

Section 1: Breast: Pathological and Surgical Approach

1. Pathological Approach 3
   Maria Sotiropoulou
2. Surgical Approach 11
   Constantine Dimitrakakis

Section 2: Basic Principles of Elastography

3. Elastography and Tissue Strain: What Clinicians Need to Know 15
   Christina An. Gkali

Section 3: Strain Imaging: Basic Principles and Examination Protocol

4. Strain Imaging 21
   Christina An. Gkali
5. Strain Imaging Examination Protocol 30
   Christina An. Gkali

Section 4: Acoustic Radiation Force Impulse Imaging: Basic Principles and Examination Protocol

6. Acoustic Radiation Force Impulse Imaging 35
   Christina An. Gkali
7. Acoustic Radiation Force Impulse Imaging Examination Protocol 49
   Christina An. Gkali

Section 5: Suggested Breast Ultrasound Elastography Reporting

8. Breast Ultrasound Elastography Reporting 55
   Christina An. Gkali

Section 6: Interpretation of Benign and Malignant Breast Lesions

9. Interpretation of Benign Breast Lesions 61
   Christina An. Gkali
10. Interpretation of Malignant Breast Lesions 99
    Christina An. Gkali
11. Pitfalls 132
    Christina An. Gkali

Index *141*

SECTION 1

BREAST: PATHOLOGICAL AND SURGICAL APPROACH

CHAPTER 1

Pathological Approach

Maria Sotiropoulou

Breasts are the specialized organs of mammals for the milk production.

The shape and size of the breast depend upon age, parity and menopausal status. There are genetic and racial variations. Breasts are formed of compound tubule-alveolar glands, ducts and adipose tissue covered by thin skin with a specialized structure, the nipple. The covering skin includes areola, a central pink to pigmented area with Montgomery tubercles, which corresponding prominent sebaceous glands, and the nipple as an elevation in the center.

Several collecting ducts (approximately 20) drain a mammary lobe which opens in the nipple. The duct system below the collection duct is the lactiferous sinus (which communicates with segmental duct follow by subsegmental and finally into terminal ducts). Each lobule is an independent system and may have 20–40 lobules with acini which are the terminal part of the ductal system (Fig. 1.1).

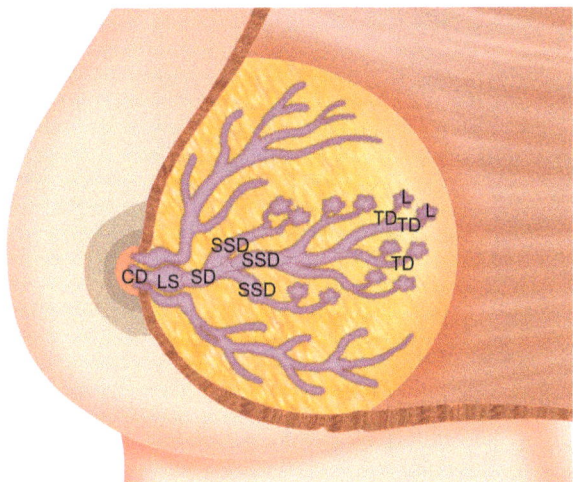

Fig. 1.1: Breast ductal system.
(CD: Central duct; LS: Lactiferous sinus; SD: Segmental duct; SSD: Subsegmental duct; TD: Terminal duct; L: Lobule).

Each lobule in normal breast consists of 10–100 acini, so the lobular unit of the breast is the terminal duct lobular unit (TDLU) from which originates the most benign and malignant breast processes. So diseases arise from the TDLU are cysts, epithelial hyperplasia, intraductal and invasive carcinoma, while from lactiferous, segmental and subsegmental ducts the solitary intraductal papilloma and ductal ectasia (Fig. 1.2).

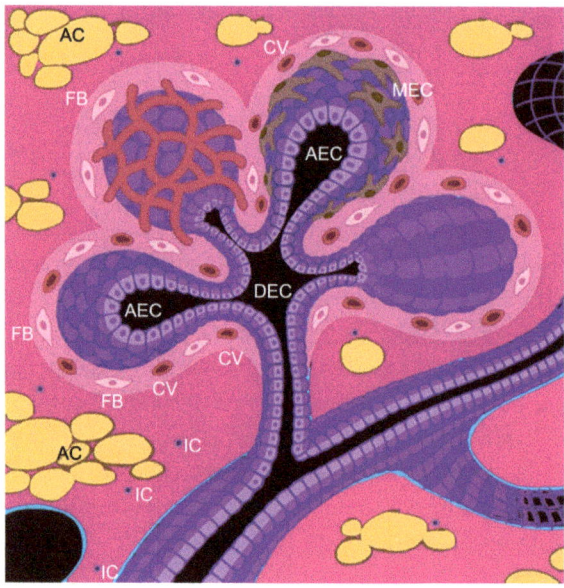

Fig. 1.2: Terminal ductal lobular unit (TDLU).
(DEC: Ductal epithelial cell; AEC: Alveolar epithelial cell; MEC: Myoepithelial cell; FB: Fibroblast; CV: Capillary vessel; IC: Immune cell; AC: Adipose cell).

The whole parenchymal tree is lined luminal by cuboidal or low columnar epithelial cells surrounded by a distinct layer of myoepithelial cells. Columnar cells have plentiful organelles and were involved in the secretion while the basal-myoepithelial cells of the lobules and ducts have a role in milk flow during lactation. The lobules embedded in a specialized loose connective stroma within which sparse of lymphocytes or plasma cells, histiocytes and mast cells are often present (Fig. 1.3).

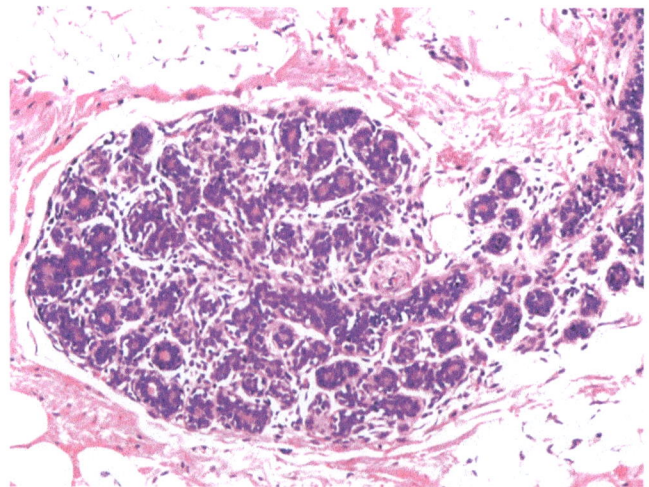

Fig. 1.3: Terminal ductal lobular unit (TDLU) with acini and subsegmental duct (H&E x200).

The luminal cells usually express low molecular weight cytokeratins (LMW-CKs) like CK7, CK8, CK18 and CK19. The majority expresses estrogen receptor-alpha (ER-α), progesterone receptors (PgRs) and androgen receptors (ARs) as a heterogeneous pattern. The myoepithelial cells have epithelial and myoid phenotype and express "basic" high molecular weight cytokeratins (HMW-CKs) CK5/5, CK14, CK17 and molecules as calponin, smooth muscle myosin heavy chain (SMM-HC), smooth muscle actin and type IV collagen while do not express ER-α, AR and PgR (Fig. 1.4).

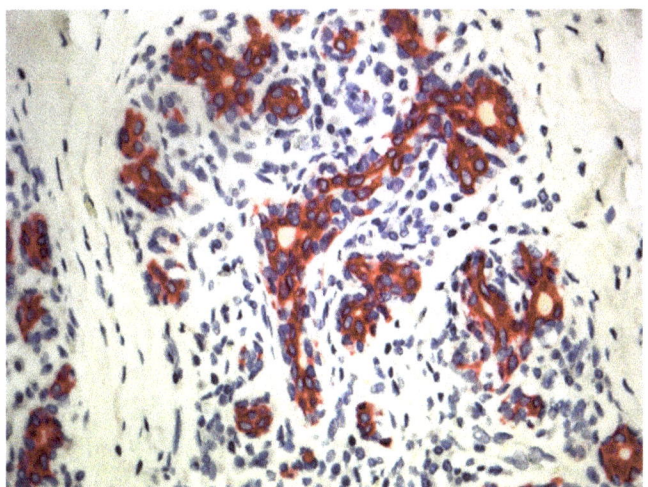

Fig. 1.4: Terminal ductal lobular unit (TDLU): Myoepithelial cells with immunohistochemical stain CK5/6 (x400).

Terminal duct lobular units are surrounded by loose connective tissue with no elastic fibers while later is present along the length of duct system. Women after the age of 50 have abundant elastic tissue in the periductal stroma. Marked periductal elastic fiber deposition was found in less than 3% of young women breast and in 17% in women older than age 50. The whole of stromal and epithelial components and the amount of each reflect the radiographic appearance between normal and pathologic conditions.

The histology of the breast is subject to changes in the menstrual cycle, pregnancy, lactation, hormone administration and menopause. With the onset of puberty, the breast starts developing by elongation of ducts and thickening of the epithelium on the one hand and the differentiation of the surrounded stroma on the second hand, due to the secretion of estrogen and progesterone by the ovaries. The maturation of breast occurs with the onset of puberty but progresses a decade later and completed mainly in pregnancy. Cellular and structural changes that occur in the mammary gland during the cycle described in detail by Vogel et al. During follicular phase, the breast has the lower parenchymal density while in luteal phase the breast increases in volume due to increase water content. In proliferative phase, there is increase in mitoses and apoptotic bodies of epithelial cells. The lobular stroma is dense and hypovascular with fibroblasts surrounded as a ring around lobular glands.

Mitotic activity is decreased in the follicular phase while lobular stroma is edematous. During pregnancy, there is enlargement of lobules and relative decreased fibrofatty stroma. With the beginning of pregnancy, terminal ducts and lobules proliferate and increase stromal vascularity with participation mononuclear leukocytes. The myoepithelial cells become blurred due to the great proliferation of epithelial cells (Fig. 1.5). Breast complete involution happens 3 months after the end of lactation. The collagen-rich fibrous tissue is higher in young women and is responsible for the density of the breast which is most pronounced in young.

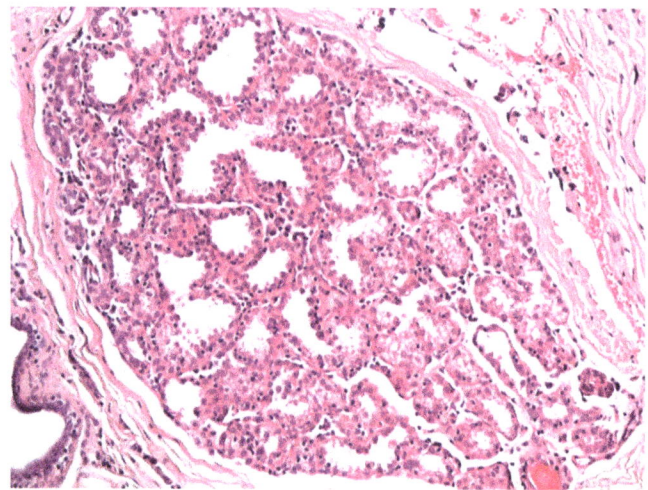

Fig. 1.5: Lactating breast: lobular hyperplasia with distended acini (H&E x200).

The breast is the target organ of a variety of hormones especially estrogen and progesterone. The proportion of the hormone receptors in the breast varies in the phases of the menstrual cycle. During pregnancy, role of development has not only ER and PgR but also prolactin, steroids, insulin and growth hormone. The percentage of ER and PgR (nuclear stain) is higher in lobular than ductal cells and is approximately 7% in normal breast cells. After menopause, ER-positive cells increase and the expression is in a continuous pattern (Figs. 1.6A and B). The high expression rate there is in late proliferative and luteal phases while decreases during pregnancy and lactation.

The invasive carcinoma of the breast derived from a series of intermediate progress or proliferative stages (with or without atypia) and neoplastic conditions such as intraepithelial carcinoma. Molecular and genetic studies in breast have problems in estimation because of morphological heterogeneity of epithelial preinvasive lesions and the surrounded environment (adipose tissue, blood components, lymph vessels, inflammatory cells). Epithelial cells of normal terminal tubule-lobular units and hyperplastic ones have the same morphology while proliferation index is two to three times greater. At the same time, the expression of ER is increased until 80–90% in atypical ductal hyperplasia. The molecular changes in the intraductal carcinoma [ductal carcinoma in situ (DCIS)] depend on the nuclear grade and proliferation index

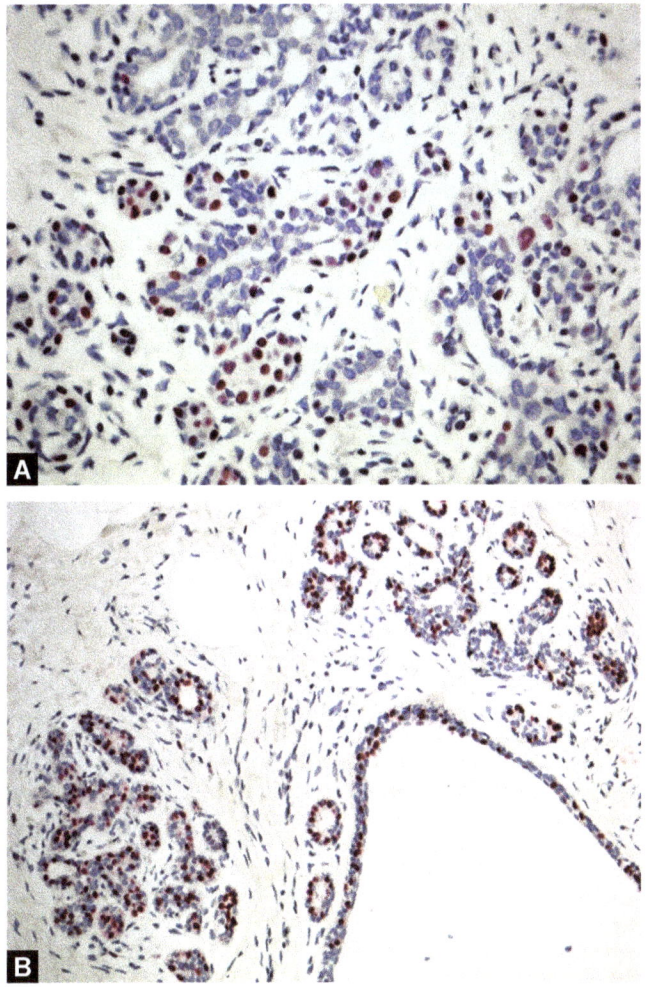

Figs. 1.6A and B: Lobule with immunostain for estrogen receptor (ER). (A) Premenopausal breast (H&E x400); (B) Higher percentage in postmenopausal breast (H&E x200).

(Ki67), the latter is two to ten times more than normal epithelium. Human epidermal growth factor receptor-2 (HER-2), that is implicated in target therapy, is a membrane tyrosine kinase oncogene that is amplified and overexpresses in the protein level in about 20% of invasive breast cancer and in 50–75% in high-grade DCIS. In contrary, lobular neoplasia has low proliferation index and negative HER-2. Circulating estrogens acting on the breast epithelium binds and stimulates the nuclear transcription factor ER-α which then adjusted the composition of PgR. ER-α-positive proliferating cells are few in normal epithelium while in hyperplastic units are five times more. Differences can be found in apoptosis in normal units related to hyperplastic ones (apoptotic index 0.61 and 0.22 respectively). The estrogen receptor-beta (ER-β) is not necessary for the development of breast ducts but inhibits the action of ER-α after conversion into heterodimers. Tumor cells exist genetic alterations of oncogenes, mutations and deactivation suppressor genes, point mutations, loss of heterozygosity, aneuploidy, and rearranging chromosomes. The loss of heterozygosity observed in normal nontumor structures adjacent to invasive breast carcinoma.

Carcinogenesis occurs with both the paths one hand "immortalization" due to loss of tumor suppressor pathways which intervenes in regulating the cell cycle and apoptosis, and other hand oncogenesis, this additional genetic changes that lead to the development of active capacity regardless of microenvironment limitations. In previous decades, there was the epitheliocentric perception of carcinogenesis which is replaced today by the theory that the growth of a tumor due to the interaction between stroma and epithelium. Epigenetic model supports that the microenvironment exerts an initial inhibitory effect. Extracellular matrix and the myoepithelium can regulate the bioavailability of growth factors and inhibit angiogenesis. Neoplastic conversion of epithelial cells disrupts the homeostatic regulation leading to disturbance of architectural cohesion. The inherited genetic changes predisposing to malignancy increasing the risk with reduced penetrance, modify the risk associated with other genes or environmental factors, are involved in repairs of deoxyribonucleic acid (DNA), are creating genetic instability, are involved in cell death, survival, proliferation, invasiveness, mobility and drug resistance. Breast carcinogenesis and invasiveness are involved by stromal cells, fibroblasts and immunity cells as the lymphocytes infiltrated the tumor. The stroma accompanying breast tumors contains an increased number of fibroblasts and immune cells, enhanced capillary density, increased collagen I and fibrin deposition. All these can alter the structure of the extracellular matrix and induce changes in the adjacent epithelium. The tumor-associated stroma shows elevated expression of alpha-smooth muscle actin (α-SMA), collagen IV, prolyl 4-hydroxylase, fibroblast-activated protein (FAP), tenascin, desmin, calponin, etc. The tumor microenvironment involved the stiffness of tissue with involvement of extracellular matrix and beta-1 integrin/phosphoinositide 3-kinase (PI3K) pathway.

In recent years, there are dramatic changes in pathology of the breast cancer diagnosis and treatment. Consequently, there is a rapid increase of necessity for specialties related to breast cancer to communicate each other. There are available many imaging techniques which one hand will help in the diagnosis and the other part in making the appropriate biopsy. Mammography remains the main tool for the detection of breast cancer assisted by other imaging methods highlight ultrasound.

The breast density reflects the percentage of glandular elements in relation of adipose tissue and divided into four grades: (1) fatty, (2) scattered, (3) intermediate and (4) dense. An attractive feature of tumor microenvironment is the tumor-associated tissue stiffness. The tissue rigidity is clinically known as an oncogenic risk factor correlated with dense breast. In addition, tumor stiffness is one of characteristics that clinicians look for, during palpation of patients who suspect breast cancer. Ultrasonography is pivotal additional aid in the detection and the determination of the importance of palpable breast lesions. The American College of Radiologists applies the ultrasound terminology lexicon Breast Imaging Reporting and Data System (BI-RADS) to standard breast lesions depending on the risk be a malignancy. It is proved that the BI-RADS 3 category has chance of malignancy only 2% nevertheless leads to close monitoring and unnecessary biopsies with high financial and psychological implications. The hardness of breast lesions is closely associated with the degree of malignancy and is the basis of the evaluation the possibility of malignancy by elastography. The application of the elastic sonography which is based on the stiffness of a distortion appeared to restrict the BI-RADS category. The firmness of the tissues regulated by the relationship between the cells of the extracellular matrix and in general tumor microenvironment and is affected partly by desmoplastic reaction which is observed in infiltration of surrounding tissues by malignant tumors. The increased stiffness also correlates with the level of aggression in breast cancer based on Bloom-Richardson histological grading system, size, lymph node involvement, lymphangiogenesis and vascular invasion. The pioneer studies conducted by Perou and Sørlie reported a distinctive molecular portrait of breast cancer using 456 cDNA clones according to which tumors were classified into five intrinsic subtypes with clinical outcomes: (1) luminal A, (2) luminal B, (3) HER-2 overexpression, (4) basal and (5) normal like tumors. Recent studies have shown a correlation between the breast stiffness measured by ultrasound shear elastography and luminal A and luminal B subtypes linked with cell proliferation marker—Ki67 and histologic grade. Moreover, triple negative (ER, PgR, HER-2) and HER-2-positive breast cancer subtypes were showed greater stiffness than ER-positive tumors. All breast cancers classified as BI-RADS 3 on B-mode ultrasound were triple negative.

In conclusion, histology of the epithelium and microenvironment of the breast lesions associated with the stiffness in which the elastography based, moreover BI-RADS terminology correlates with histological and molecular factors and clinical prognostic parameters.

SUGGESTED READING

Arendt LM, Rudnick JA, Keller PJ, et al. Stroma in breast development and disease. Semin Cell Dev Biol. 2010;21(1):11-8.
Bernstein L, Press M. Does estrogen receptor expression in normal breast tissue predict breast cancer risk? J Natl Cancer Inst. 1998;90(1):5-7.
Boyd NF, Li Q, Melnichouk O, et al. Evidence that breast tissue stiffness is associated with risk of breast cancer. PloS One. 2014;9(7):e100937.
Chang JM, Park IA, Lee SH, et al. Stiffness of tumors measured by shear-wave elastography correlated with subtypes of breast cancer. Eur Radiol. 2013;23(9):2450-8.
Cha YJ, Youk JH, Kim BG, et al. Lymphangiogenesis in breast cancer correlates with matrix stiffness on shear-wave elastography. Yonsei Med J. 2016;57(3):599-605.
Collins LC, Schnitt SJ. Breast. Stacey ME (Ed). Histology for Pathologists, 4th edition. Philadelphia: Lippincott Williams & Wilkins; 2012. p. 67.
Cukierman E. A visual-quantitative analysis of fibroblastic stromagenesis in breast cancer progression. J Mammary Gland Biol Neoplasia. 2004;9:311-24.
Deng G, Lu Y, Zlotnikov G, et al. Loss of heterozygosity in normal tissue adjacent to breast carcinomas. Science. 1996;274:2057-9,.
Denis M, Gregory A, Bayat M, et al. Correlating tumor stiffness with immunohistochemical subtypes of breast cancers: prognostic value of comb-push ultrasound shear elastography for differentiating luminal subtypes. PloS One. 2016;11:e0165003.
Evans A, Whelehan P, Thomson K, et al. Differentiating benign from malignant breast masses: value of shear wave elastography according to lesion stiffness combined with grayscale ultrasound according to BI-RADS classification. Br J Cancer. 2012;107:224-9.
Evans A, Whelehan P, Thomson K, et al. Invasive breast cancer relationship between shear-wave elastographic findings and histologic prognostic factors. Radiology. 2012;263(3):673-7.

Hanahan D, Weinberg RA. Hallmarks of cancer: next generation. Cell. 2011;144:646-74.

Hayashi M, Yamamoto Y, Sueta A, et al. Associations between elastography findings and clinicopathological factors in breast cancer. Medicine (Baltimore). 2015;94(50):e2290.

Hoda SA. Anatomy and physiologic morphology. Hoda SA, Brogi E, Koerner FC, Rosen PP (Eds). Rosen's Breast Pathology, 4th edition. Philadelphia: Lippincott Williams & Wilkins; 2014.

Hoda SA. Normal breast and developmental disorders. Dabbs DJ (Ed). Breast Pathology, 1st edition. Philadelphia: Elsevier; 2012.

Perou CM, Sørlie T, Eisen MB, et al. Molecular portraits of human breast tumors. Nature. 2000;406:747-52.

Pickup MW, Mouw JK, Weaver VM. The extracellular matrix modulates the hallmarks of cancer. EMBO Rep. 2014;15:1243-53.

Shaaban AM, Sloane JP, West CR, et al. Breast cancer risk in usual ductal hyperplasia is defined by estrogen receptor-alpha and Ki-67 expression. Am J Pathol. 2002;160(2):597-604.

Vogel PM, Georgiade NG, Fetter BF, et al. The correlation of histologic changes in the human breast with the menstrual cycle. Am J Pathol. 1981;104:23-34.

CHAPTER 2

Surgical Approach

Constantine Dimitrakakis

Breast cancer is the most common cancer in women worldwide. There are many risk factors responsible for increasing the chance of developing breast cancer. Some of them can be modified, whereas most of them cannot be influenced. Among the nonmodifiable risk factors are age, gender (female), genetic risk factors (mainly mutations in the BRCA1 and the BRCA2), family history (first-degree relative with breast cancer), personal history of breast, ovarian, or endometrial cancer, personal history of lymphoma and chest radiation, early menarche, late menopause, breast density, long-term or high-dose estrogen replacement therapy. Factors that can be modified are obesity, alcohol, use of female hormones and physical exercise.

Breast screening and early diagnosis of breast cancer is very important in successful treatment management. Early diagnosis prolongs women's life and develops quality of life. It becomes obvious that the cornerstone of breast cancer confrontation and at the same time the biggest challenge is the early detection of malignant breast lesions that ensures a timely and effective treatment. On the other hand, it is also of crucial importance to reduce unnecessary biopsies that result in increased financial cost and patient anxiety. Although mammography remains the standard for breast cancer screening, there are limitations that affect the method's sensitivity and specificity. Specifically, sensitivity in dense breasts has been reported to be as low as 30–48%. A good proportion of women at any age, as well as relatively young women, present with dense breasts where mammography, even digital, has low detection rates. In the era of an increased incidence of breast cancer in younger women, an imaging method complementary to mammography becomes urgently required. Nowadays, with the vast development in ultrasound machines, breast ultrasound is not only used to differentiate cystic from solid masses. However, a substantial overlap of benign and malignant breast lesions have been shown according to their sonographic features.

Breast Imaging Reporting and Data System (BI-RADS) is used in imaging to identify and classify breast lesions according to the possibility of the lesion to be malignant. However, BI-RADS reporting may lead to confusion in breast imaging interpretations. In particular, in BI-RADS category 4, a large proportion of patients undergo invasive diagnostic procedures that might not be necessary, if better imaging methods were available for accurate diagnosis. In contrast, in BI-RADS category 3, some malignant lesions escape early diagnosis and a complementary method could be helpful.

Breast biopsy remains the gold standard for definitive diagnosis of breast lesions and a large number of diagnostic procedures are being used as an adjunct to other imaging modalities to differentiate benign from malignant breast lesions. The pathological result is benign in up to 75% of all cases, and according to Chiou et al., the rate of cancer detection in biopsies is just 10–30%. Therefore, a reliable, noninvasive, cost-effective method that could reduce the number of unnecessary interventional diagnostic procedures would be valuable.

Several imaging techniques are currently being investigated to find the most reliable and consistent method for diagnosis of breast lesions. Ultrasound elastography is a relatively new promising method that has been used since 2003 as a helpful adjunct tool to ultrasonography. The main advantage of ultrasound elastography versus ultrasonography is that it can identify benign and malignant breast lesions based on their tissue elasticity. Thus, it seems to improve accuracy in diagnosis of breast cancer. It can reduce the unnecessary biopsies in BI-RADS 4 breast lesions and increase the malignant detection rate in BI-RADS 3 category.

In the following chapters two types of elastography, Strain and Acoustic Radiation Force Impulse (both Virtual Touch Tissue Imaging and Virtual Touch Quantification) will be presented covering a wide range of breast pathologies.

SUGGESTED READING

Chiou SY, Chou YH, Chiou HJ, et al. Sonographic features of nonpalpable breast cancer: a study based on ultrasound-guided wire-localized surgical biopsies. Ultrasound Med Biol. 2006;32(9);1299-306.

D'Orsi CJ, Sickles EA, Mendelson EB, et al. ACR BI-RADS® Atlas, Breast Imaging Reporting and Data System. Reston, VA, American College of Radiology; 2013

Kolb TM, Lichy J, Newhouse JH. Comparison of the performance of screening mammography, physical examination, and breast US and evaluation of factors that influence them: an analysis of 27,825 patient evaluations. Radiology. 2002;225(1):165-75.

Mandelson MT, Oestreicher N, Porter PL, et al. Breast density as a predictor of mammographic detection: Comparison of interval- and screen-detected cancers. J Natl Cancer Inst. 2000;92(13):1081-7.

Moon WK, Chang SC, Huang CS, et al. Breast tumor classification using fuzzy clustering for breast elastography. Ultrasound Med Bio. 2011;37(5):700-8.

Rahbar G, Sie AC, Hansen GC, et al. Benign versus malignant solid breast masses: US differentiation. Radiology. 1999;213(3):889-94.

Siegel R, Naishadham D, Jemal A. CA Cancer J Clin. 2013; 63(1):11-30.

SECTION 2

BASIC PRINCIPLES OF ELASTOGRAPHY

CHAPTER 3

Elastography and Tissue Strain: What Clinicians Need to Know

Christina An. Gkali

Ultrasound imaging is a first-line imaging modality for a wide range of indications, playing a major role in screening, diagnosis, and therapeutic interventions for various diseases and pathologies. However, even with enormous improvements in recent years, conventional ultrasound is limited in its ability to differentiate between the mechanical properties of tissue, which can be important in assessing the morphology and physiology of focal or diffuse disease.

Ultrasound elastography was initially introduced as a new imaging method adjunct to ultrasound in order to overcome ultrasonography limitations, such as increased number of unnecessary biopsies.

The system which was used for all the cases described in this book was a Siemens Acuson S2000. The techniques that we are going to describe are strain imaging and acoustic radiation force impulse (ARFI) based on our equipment.

Compression elastography offered the promise of a new dimension of ultrasound. In addition to the anatomic detail visible in B-mode and the flow imaging offered by color Doppler, elastography was intended to enable visualization of tissue stiffness, long known as a harbinger of disease and malignancy (palpation searches for stiffness, after all). Early compression elastography could provide relative, qualitative visualization of tissue stiffness differences for assessing focal lesions, but lacked the ability to quantify stiffness differences of these lesions.

Acoustic radiation force impulse technology allows to enable both qualitative and quantitative assessment of the mechanical stiffness (elasticity) differences in tissue. Ultrasound systems can be configured with a wide range of elastography technologies and applications, helping physicians evaluate conditions of the liver, breast, thyroid and other organs.

ELASTOGRAPHY AND TISSUE STRAIN

The perfect diagnostic tool would have 100% sensitivity (a positive result when disease is present) and 100% specificity (a negative result in the absence of disease) in all cases. Such a technology does not exist, of course. However, the use of more than one imaging tool can provide overall higher diagnostic accuracy than one imaging modality alone. This is true when adding elastography to conventional ultrasound and when using multiple elastography technologies in cooperation.

Modern elastography can refer to multiple technologies. Some depend upon heavy user-generated manual pressure. More advanced elasticity imaging, enabled by sophisticated architecture, can detect extremely small changes in tissue displacements (on the order of 1–10 μm). These advanced elastography tools rely less on manual pressure and can detect tissue stiffness based on native tissue motion, induced by the patient's cardiac pulsations and respiration.

Using ARFI technology, rather than manual compression techniques, tissue is compressed by an acoustic beam. One advantage of this approach is that the acoustic beam is focused at the region of interest (ROI) to maximize the local displacement of tissue, rather than just at the skin surface with uncontrollable stress being applied in deeper tissues. This more controllable application of stress improves the uniformity of the resulting elastogram.

Acoustic radiation force impulse technology also induces and tracks the propagation of shear waves (transverse waves) for quantification of tissue stiffness. An increase in shear wave velocity correlates closely with increasing tissue stiffness, providing a more precise indication of true tissue elasticity at a point location.

This ability to quantify tissue stiffness, rather than qualitatively evaluating stiffness compared to surrounding tissue with focal lesions, expands the clinical utility of elastography to homogeneous tissue, such as liver and spleen.

In addition, compared to manual compression, ARFI offers a reduction in user technique dependence. The user simply initiates the acquisition of the elastogram or quantitative measurement with the push of a button, further improving interoperator reproducibility, which is an important aspect of clinical utility (Figs. 3.1A to C).

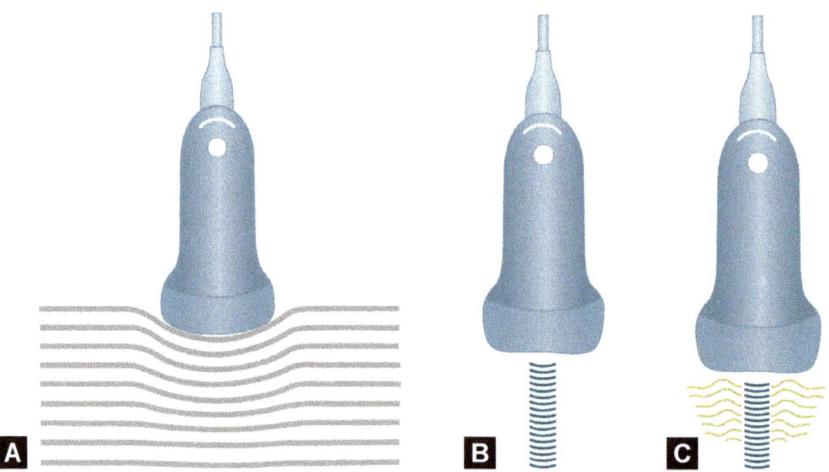

Figs. 3.1A to C: Elastography technologies attributed schematically. (A) Compression elastography; (B) Acoustic radiation force impulse (ARFI) elastography; (C) Shear wave detection for quantification at a single point.

HOW ELASTOGRAPHY WORKS

Physics of Tissue Strain

Many studies have characterized the normal range of elasticity values of various tissue types and that certain disease processes can change the viscoelastic properties of tissue. Elastography tools work by measuring how much strain tissues exhibit in response to stress. The relationship between stress and strain provides information about the mechanical stiffness of the tissue in question.

Stress and strain are not the same. Stress is the force exerted and strain is what happens to the tissue in response to the pressure.

Two kinds of strain exist, longitudinal and shear, as shown in Figures 3.2A and B.

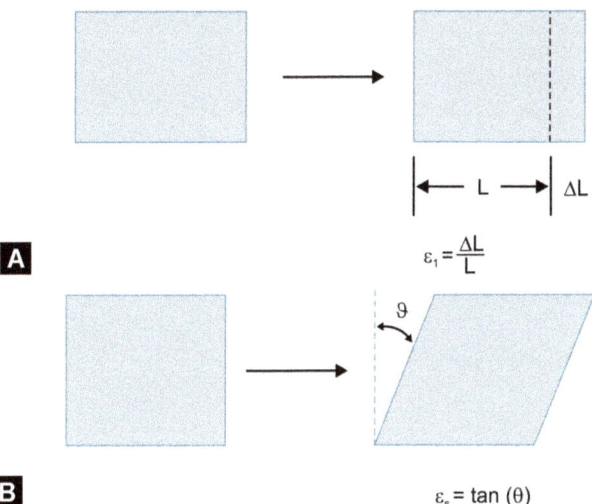

Figs. 3.2A and B: (A) Longitudinal strain; (B) Shear strain.

Longitudinal, or normal strain, occurs when tissue is either stretched or compressed. Shear strain occurs as a result of angular forces, such as twisting or bending.

In tissue, both longitudinal and shear strains are usually present when manual compression force or radiation force is used. In fluid, pressure is the same in all directions; therefore, shear strain and shear waves do not exist in fluids.

Hooke's law describes the relationship between stress and strain for most materials, including viscoelastic tissue:

$$\sigma = Y\varepsilon$$

where

σ is a deformation proportional to the force of ε.

Young's modulus or modulus of elasticity can be computed by examining the slope of the stress/strain diagram in the elastic portion of the curve, as shown in Figure 3.3.

The shear modulus G, also known as the modulus of rigidity, can also be calculated through examination of a shear stress versus shear strain curve.

In elastic materials, the relationship between the velocity of a shear wave and shear modulus is:

$$v_s = \sqrt{\frac{G}{\rho}}$$

where G is the tissue shear modulus and ρ is the solid tissue density.

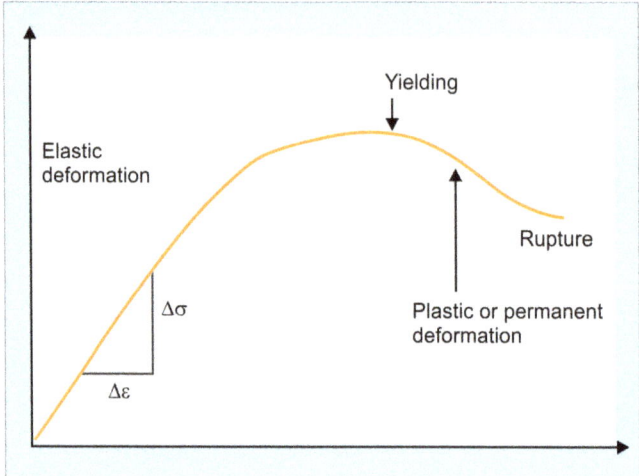

Fig. 3.3: Relationship between strain and stress in any material.

Tissues with a higher shear modulus, or modulus of rigidity (less compliant to shear forces), will have a higher shear wave velocity than tissues with a lower modulus of rigidity (more compliant to shear forces).

SUGGESTED READING

Rosen J, Brown J, De S, Sinanan M, Hannford B. Biomechanical Properties of Abdominal Organs In Vivo and Postmortem Under Compression Loads. Journal of Biomechanical Engineering. 2008; Vol. 130, 021020-1.

Wellman, et. al. Breast Tissue Stiffness in Compression is Correlated to Histological Diagnosis. Harvard BioRobotics Laboratory Technical Report, 1999. https://biorobotics. harvard.edu/pubs/1999/mechprops.pdf.

SECTION 3

STRAIN IMAGING: BASIC PRINCIPLES AND EXAMINATION PROTOCOL

CHAPTER 4 | Strain Imaging

Christina An. Gkali

With strain imaging (eSie Touch elasticity, Siemens Healthcare), the elastogram is created using either minimal compression or physiologic tissue motion from cardiac pulsations or respiration as the stress force on tissue (Fig. 4.1). Compressive strain of tissue is recorded in the image through continuous analysis of acquired ultrasonic detection signals.

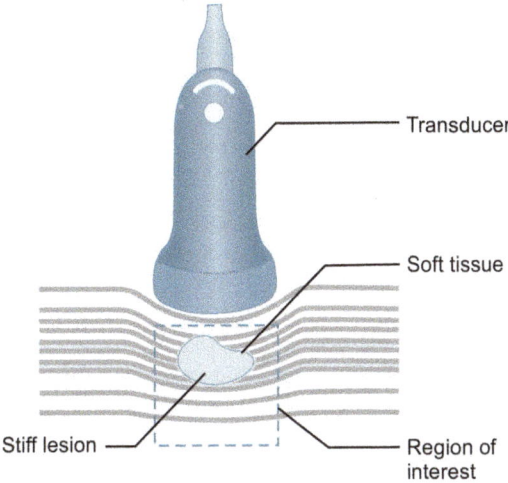

Fig. 4.1: With eSie Touch elasticity imaging, tissue strain is induced by minimal mechanical compression with the transducer or cardiac pulsations and respiration.

Detection pulses track displacement, which are used to derive a strain image in grayscale (Figs. 4.2 and 4.3) or color-coded display (Fig. 4.4).

■ STRAIN IMAGE IN GRAYSCALE

Pathology result was suggestive of fibroadenoma.
 The grayscale map at the side shows that the darker the lesion is the higher the stiffness is.
 Pathology result was suggestive of ductal adenocarcinoma grade III with foci of ductal carcinoma in situ (DCIS) grade III and microcalcifications.

■ QUALITATIVE EVALUATION OF GRAYSCALE STRAIN IMAGE

Visual evaluation of grayscale strain image is feasible with a grayscale map according to which the darker the lesion is the higher the stiffness (compared to the surrounding tissue). The grayscale map appears besides to the dual B-mode and strain image.

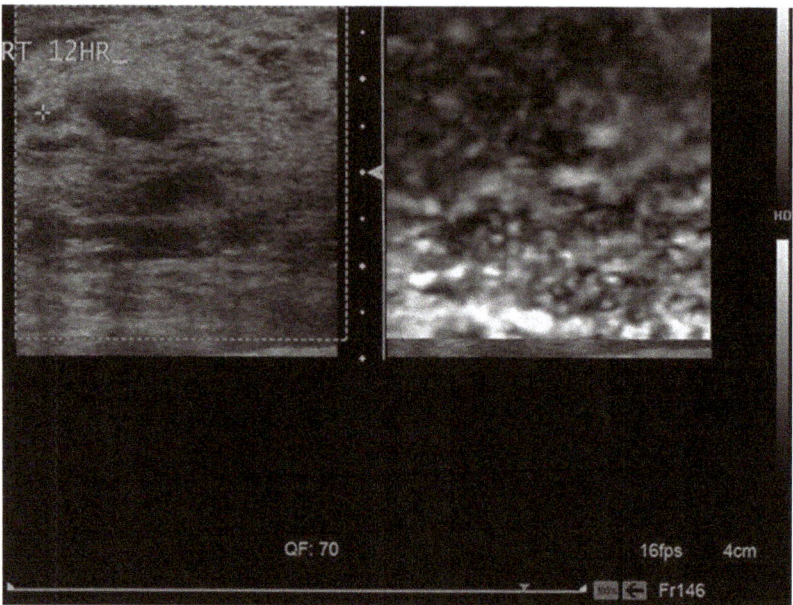

Fig. 4.2: Dual image of B-mode and grayscale strain image of an oval, well-defined, hypoechoic breast lesion. The lesion is depicted as dark as the surrounding tissue in the grayscale strain image (same stiffness).

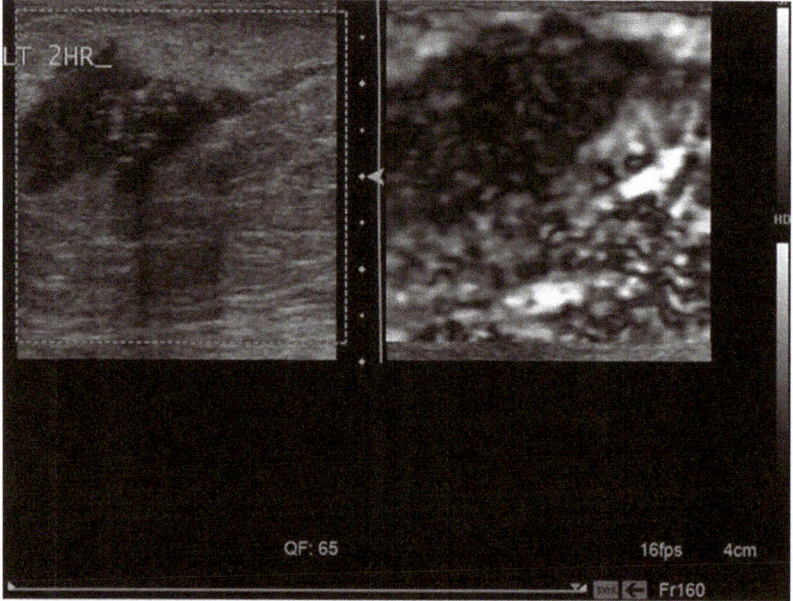

Fig. 4.3: Dual image of B-mode and grayscale strain image of a marked hypoechoic, with irregular, ill-defined margins and presence of calcifications. The lesion appears marked darker than the surrounding tissue in the grayscale strain image. The darker the lesion is depicted in grayscale strain image compared to surrounding tissue, the stiffer the lesion is.

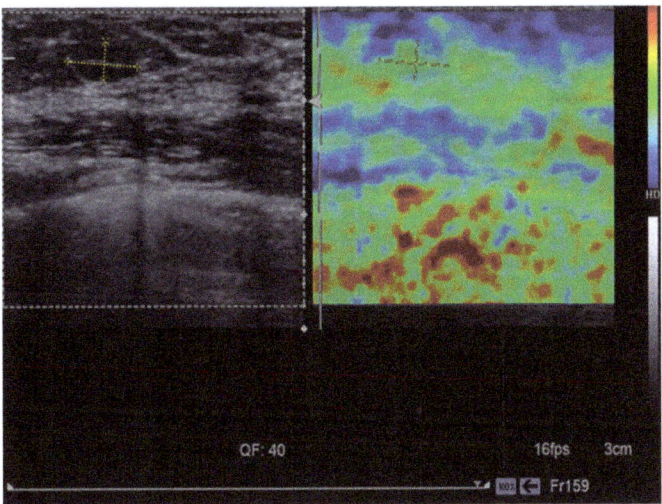

Fig. 4.4: Dual image of B-mode and color map strain image of a biopsy-proven fibroadenoma. B-mode depicts an oval, well-defined, hypoechoic mass which appears green in color map strain image, which means that the lesion is soft.

A lesion size on elastography to the B-mode size ratio was proposed as a diagnostic tool to differentiate benign from malignant breast lesions. This ratio is named EI/B ratio.

According to the literature lesions with EI/B ratio greater than or less than 1 are considered to be malignant, whereas lesions with EI/B ratio less than 1 benign (Fig. 4.5). An EI/B ratio greater than or less than 1 means that the lesion appears bigger on grayscale strain image than the B-mode image.

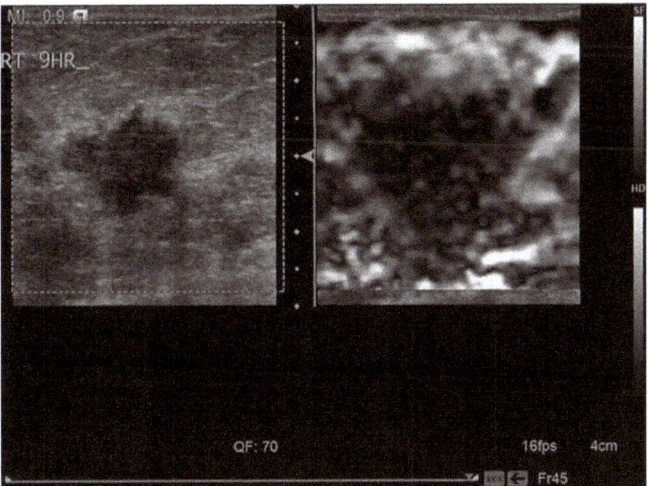

Fig. 4.5: The hypoechoic, ill-defined, spiculated mass appears larger on strain image than the B-mode corresponding image, which means EI/B ratio greater than 1 (probably malignant). The lesion is also darker than the surrounding tissue (grayscale map).

Pathology result was invasive ductal carcinoma grade III.

Hall, Zhu et al. 2003 showed that malignant lesions appear larger than the corresponding B-mode image.

Barr, Destounis et al. 2012 using an EI/B ratio greater than or less than 1 for malignant lesions showed that the sensitivity and specificity is 99% and 87%, respectively.

SEMIQUANTITATIVE WAY OF STIFFNESS EVALUATION

Strain Ratio

Strain ratio is a semi-quantitative way to evaluate the stiffness of a breast lesion compared to fat (Fig. 4.6).

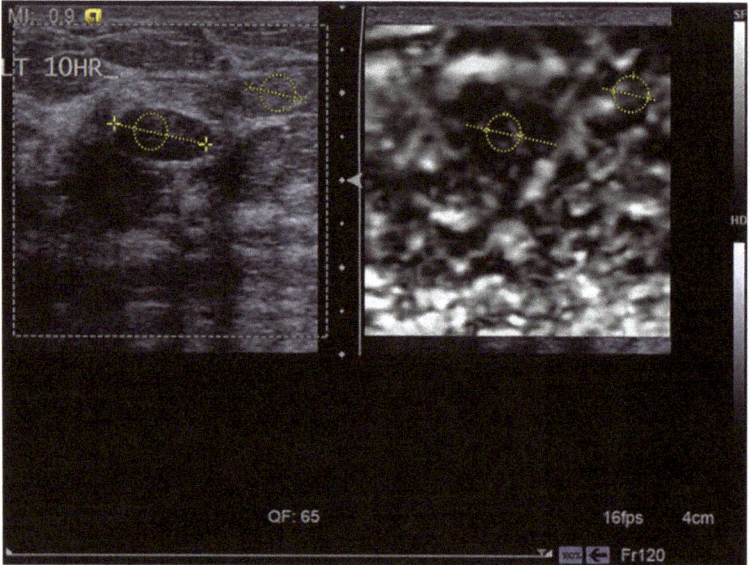

Fig. 4.6: Elastogram from a 43-year-old woman with a biopsy-proven fibroadenoma. The strain ratio is calculated by determining the ratio of the strain from the lesion compared to that of fat and is equal to 1.97, i.e. the lesion is 1.97 times stiffer than fat.

A measure of the true strain (displacement %) of all pixels in each region of interest (ROI) is obtained and a numerical value for relative stiffness displayed.

The percentage displacement for each ROI is displayed and the strain ratio is calculated. The lesion strain ratio increases as the lesion stiffness increases.

When performing strain ratio measurements, the two ROI should be of equivalent size and also positioned at approximately the same level (depth) within the image. Also, the target ROI for subcutaneous fat should be limited to fat that does not contain fibroglandular breast tissue at a similar depth to the lesion.

The cut-off point for strain ratio varies from 0.5 to 4.5 in different studies.

According to Fischer et al., the sensitivity and specificity of strain ratio were 95% and 74% respectively when using a lesion to fat cut-off ratio equal to 2.27 was used.

Thomas et al. compared B-mode breast imaging reporting and data system (BI-RADS), the 5-point color scale, and the lesion-to-fat ratio in 227 breast lesions. A cut-off point of 2.45 was used based on the receiver-operating characteristic (ROC) curve to distinguish benign from malignant lesions with 90% sensitivity and 89% specificity, respectively.

Zhi et al. in a similar study compared the strain ratio and the 5-point color scale in 559 breast lesions. A cut-off point of 3.05 was selected based on the ROC curve, with 92.4% sensitivity and 91.1% specificity, respectively.

Notice that the cases which will be interpreted in Part III of this book will be evaluated according to 3.05 cut-off point suggested by Zhi et al.

CYSTS

The elastographic appearance of breast cysts depends on the elastographic techniques which were used but should be accurate in establishing that the content is liquid.

Concerning to cystic lesions some highlights will be presented according to different equipment.

With Siemens equipment cysts appear with a typical bull's-eye sign (smaller size, white center, black peripheral circle) in the grayscale elastogram, as shown in Figure 4.7.

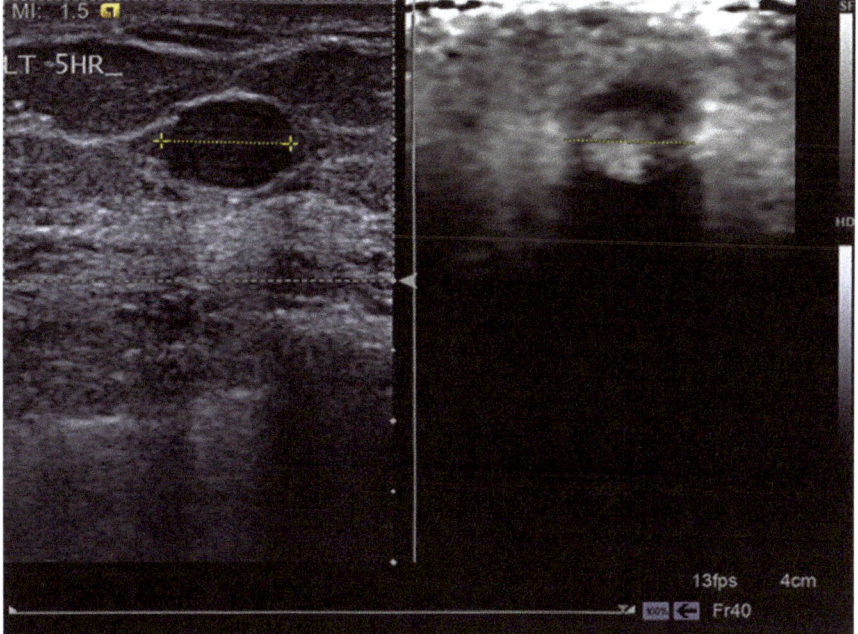

Fig. 4.7: Complicated cyst with typical bull's-eye sign.

With Hitachi and Toshiba equipment, a tri-laminar appearance of blue, green, and red (BGR) is identified in cysts (tri-color artifact).

With Philips equipment, cystic lesions have a typical three-color mixed appearance (red, green, blue) whereas with a specific software, a pure cystic content appears in yellow, and can be differentiated from a dense cyst exhibiting a blue center.

Cystic features are usually specific on elasticity imaging no internal register (acoustic radiation force impulse, Shear wave elastography).

STRAIN IMAGE IN COLOR-CODED DISPLAY

This type of color elasticity scoring uses the strain of the tissue and adds the chromatic scale assigned to the different levels of elasticity. Color mapping provides additional information about tissue stiffness. The colors may vary according to different systems and it is crucial to be aware of the one which is used. Siemens Acuson S2000 system uses red, yellow, and green to represent soft tissue whereas light and dark blue represent hard tissues.

EVALUATION OF COLOR MAPPING STRAIN IMAGE

Color map strain elastography image is visually characterized according to Tsukuba score proposed by Itoh and Ueno et al. 2006. This 5-point scale scores the lesion according to the extent of elasticity inside the lesion.

Specifically, the color map strain elastography image of a breast lesion is categorized as if follows:
- *Score* 1, when the entire lesion is deformable (green), as shown in Figure 4.8.

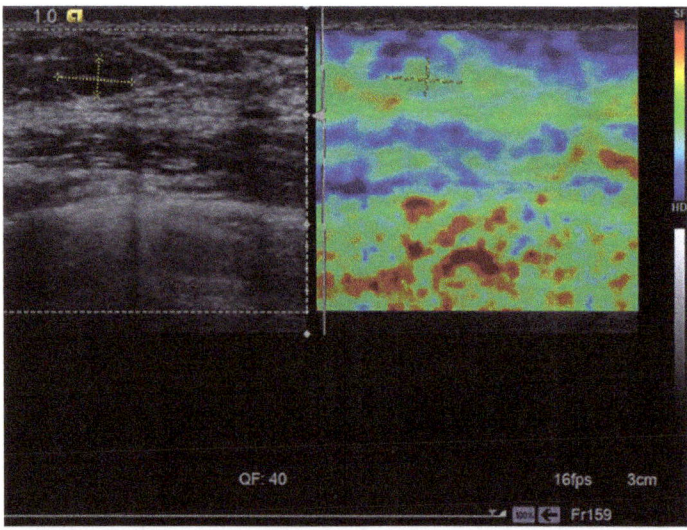

Fig. 4.8: Biopsy-proven fibroadenoma. B-mode depicts an oval, hypoechoic, well-defined mass which in color mapping is deformable (green) entirely. The elasticity score is 1.

- *Score* 2, when the most of the lesion is deformable but there are also some small stiff areas (mostly green with some blue areas), as shown in Figure 4.9.

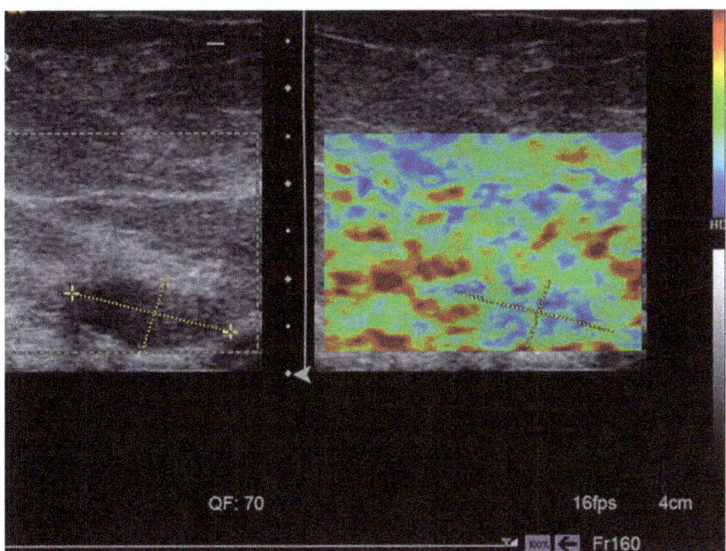

Fig. 4.9: Biopsy-proven myoepithelioma. An oval, hypoechoic mass measured 1.7 × 0.75 cm is most of its part deformable (green) with small stiff areas (blue). The elasticity score is 2.

- *Score* 3, when only the peripheral portion of the lesion is deformable with stiff tissue in the center (blue in the center and green peripherally), as shown in Figure 4.10.

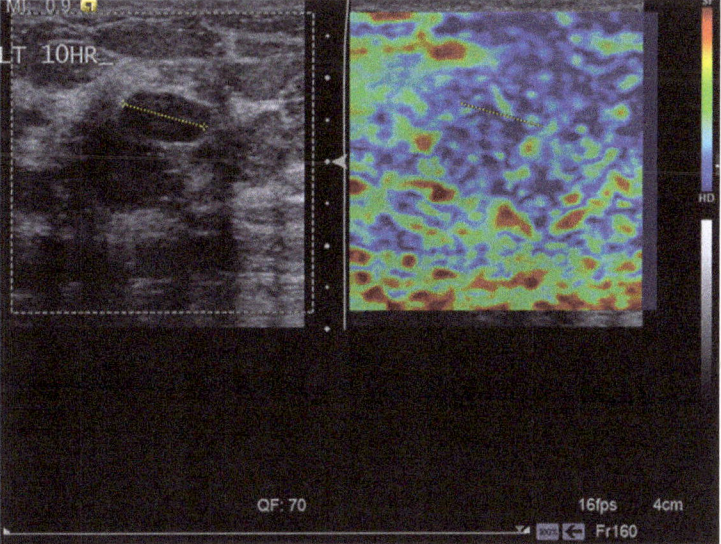

Fig. 4.10: Biopsy-proven fibroadenoma. An oval, hypoechoic mass is deformable (green) only on its peripheral part and stiff (blue) in the center. The elasticity score is 3.

- *Score* 4, when the entire lesion is stiff (blue), as shown in Figure 4.11. Pathology result was invasive ductal carcinoma grade III.

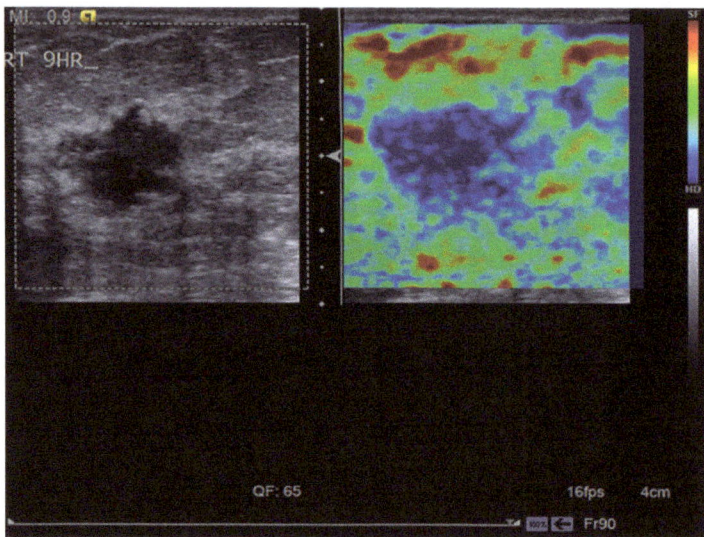

Fig. 4.11: The hypoechoic, ill-defined, spiculated mass is depicted entirely stiff (blue) in color mapping. The elasticity score is 4.

- *Score* 5, when both the entire lesion and surrounding tissue are stiff (the lesion and surrounding tissue are both blue), as shown in Figure 4.12.

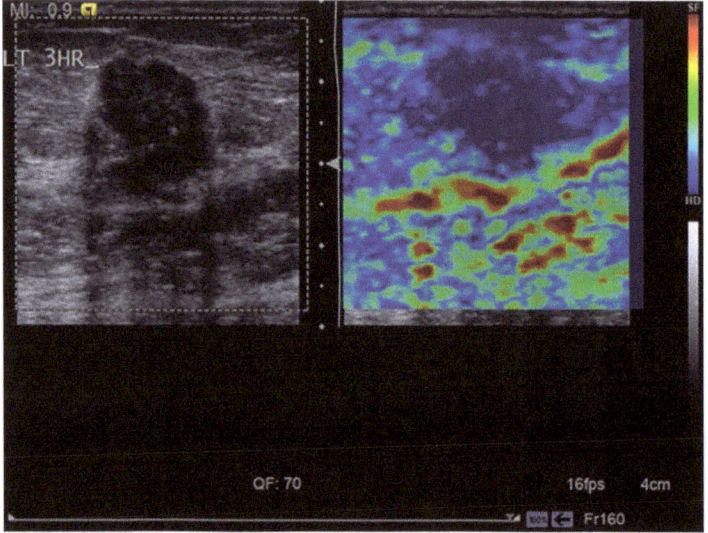

Fig. 4.12: The hypoechoic, lobulated, ill-defined mass with microcalcifications is depicted stiff as well as the surrounding tissue (blue). The elasticity score is 5.

Pathology result was ductal adenocarcinoma grade III with foci of DCIS grade III.

In a study of 111 breast lesions, Itoh and Ueno et al. showed that a cut-off point between 3 and 4 elasticity score had 86.5% sensitivity, 89.8% specificity, and 88.3% accuracy. As a result, breast lesions with Tsukuba score 1 to 3 are probably benign whereas score 4 and 5 are considered malignant.

SUGGESTED READING

Barr RG, Destounis S, Lackey LB 2nd, et al. Evaluation of breast lesions using sonographic elasticity imaging: a multicenter trial. J Ultrasound Med. 2012;31:281-7.

Barr RG, Lackey AE. The utility of the "bull's-eye" artifact on breast elasticity imaging in reducing breast lesion biopsy rate. Ultrasound Q. 2011;27:151-5.

Barr RG. Real-time ultrasound elasticity of the breast: initial clinical results. Ultrasound Q. 2010;26:61-6.

Fischer T, Peisker U, Fiedor S, et al. Significant differentiation of focal breast lesions: raw data-based calculation of strain ratio. Ultraschall Med. 2012;33:372-9.

Hall TJ, Zhu Y, Spalding CS. In vivo real-time freehand palpation imaging. Ultrasound Med Biol. 2003;29:427-43.

Itoh A, Ueno E, Tohno E, et al. Breast disease: clinical application of US elastography for diagnosis. Radiology. 2006;239:341-50.

Thomas A, Degenhardt F, Farrokh A, et al. Significant differentiation of focal breast lesions: calculation of strain ratio in breast sonoelastography. Acad Radiol. 2010;17(5):558-63.

Zhi H, Xiao XY, Yang HY, et al. Ultrasonic elastography in breast cancer diagnosis: strain ratio vs 5-point scale. Acad Radiol. 2010;10:1227-33.

CHAPTER 5
Strain Imaging Examination Protocol

Christina An. Gkali

PATIENT POSITIONING

- The patient lies on her back with her ipsilateral hand raised on the examination bed.
- The medial half of the breast is examined in the supine position.
- The lateral aspect of the breast is examined in supine oblique position (either right or left) with a foam pad positioned under the examined side of the patient.
- The patient is asked to remain and breath calmly.
- A sufficient amount of gel is applied on the skin.
- A linear transducer (4–9 MHz) is positioned perpendicular to the skin.
- The operator applies no external compression.

STRAIN ELASTOGRAPHY IMAGING

- The examination starts after positioning a linear transducer (4–9 MHz), with the B-mode image which depicts the lesion of interest, as elastography images are generated from raw data from B-mode.
- The angle of the probe should be positioned perpendicular to the skin.
- When an optimal B-mode image is obtained, strain elastography (SE) imaging is activated by using a button on the menu (it depends on the system which is used).
- The dual image of B-mode and strain image is on screen and the elastogram is observed.
- At this point, it is important to refer that if a white flash appears on the elastogram, it could be due to too much lateral movement or too little or too much pressure.
- The freeze button is pressed after approximately 10 seconds of observing.
- The cine is observed in order to obtain desired frames.
- Quality factor is an objective way to select an appropriate frame, provided by Siemens Acuson S2000 system. Higher numbers generally equate to higher quality and for breast a quality factor of greater than 55 is appropriate. But, it is of crucial meaning the quality factor to be combined with an optimal image on the elastogram.
- Then, SE-system displays tissue stiffness in a continuum of colors from green to red to blue, designating soft (high strain = green), intermediate (equal strain = red) and hard (no strain = blue) tissue (color map SE).
- Subsequently, one region of interest (ROI) is placed in the focal lesion, and the reference ROI is placed in the surrounding normal fat tissue, preferably in the same depth as the lesion. The strain ratio (SR) is automatically calculated by the elastography software.

ACQUISITION TIPS

Acquisition tips have been depicted in Box 5.1.

> **Box 5.1:** Acquisition tips.
> 1. The scan direction is optimized by positioning the patient to obtain a perpendicular plane to the chest wall.
> 2. When the lesion is located in the upper or lower outer quadrant, the patient could be turned away from the side being examined in order to bring the scan axis more perpendicular to the tissue.
> 3. The patient should remain and breath calmly. The operator's touch should be adjusted accordingly.
> 4. The region of interest (ROI) should include the area surrounding the lesion/area of interest. An image depth that allows the ROI to comprise around 50% of the total field of view is usually appropriate. The stiffness is calculated and displayed relative to the surrounding tissue.

Notification: For strain imaging, the operator has to know the best maneuver for each system and target.

There are three main types of compression methods:
1. No manual compression
2. Minimal vibration
3. Significant compression.

At this book we refer to our system which requires no manual compression.

SECTION 4

ACOUSTIC RADIATION FORCE IMPULSE IMAGING: BASIC PRINCIPLES AND EXAMINATION PROTOCOL

CHAPTER 6
Acoustic Radiation Force Impulse Imaging

Christina An. Gkali

This mode has the advantage of being objective and independent of the sonographer. Instead of using external compression, ultrasound (US) scanners are used to generate short-duration acoustic radiation forces that impart small (1–10 μm) localized displacements in the tissue. The response of the tissue to the radiation force is observed using conventional B-mode imaging pulses to track tissue displacement, which correlates with the local stiffness of the tissue. Images of tissue displacement are created by the repetition of this process along multiple image lines. A short-duration (0.03–0.4 ms), high-intensity acoustic "pushing pulse" (frequency 2.6796 MHz) in acoustic radiation force impulse (ARFI) imaging is transmitted to generate an internal tissue excitation (1–20 mm) in the region of interest (ROI) by the transducer, followed by a series of diagnostic intensity pulses (frequency 3.08 MHz, pulse repetition frequency 3–12 kHz), which are used to track the displacement of the 100 tissue caused by the pushing pulse. It is possible to display the quantitative shear wave velocity of ARFI displacement. As the velocity of the shear wave depends on tissue stiffness, it is possible to apply ARFI technology to evaluate deep tissue stiffness, which may not be possible with free-hand elastography.

On the Siemens Acuson S2000 scanner, two imaging possibilities are available.

VIRTUAL TOUCH IMAGING

Virtual touch imaging (VTI), similar to strain imaging, provides a qualitative elastogram. The VTI image depicts the relative stiffness in the selected ROI with a grayscale and also a color map. However, VTI uses ARFI instead of traditional compression or tissue motion to induce tissue displacement. VTI provides a grayscale or color-coded display of relative tissue stiffness in a user-defined ROI (Figs. 6.1 and 6.2). This information is computed by examining the displacements of tissue elements in response to an acoustic push pulse. Detection and computation of relative elasticity is similar to strain elasticity imaging.

In contrast to conventional US imaging pulsing strategy, VTI uses a three-step pulsing method.

First, a conventional US signal is acquired as a baseline in a narrow ROI.

Second, a push pulse is applied along the center of this ROI.

Third, another conventional US signal is acquired and is compared to the baseline to obtain tissue displacement.

The more elastic a given tissue element, the more displacement it experiences. This process is repeated for each axial line within the ROI, as with a conventional B-mode image.

Virtual Touch Image in Grayscale

Virtual touch image in grayscale is illustrated in Figure 6.3.

Section 4: Acoustic Radiation Force Impulse Imaging: Basic Principles and Examination Protocol

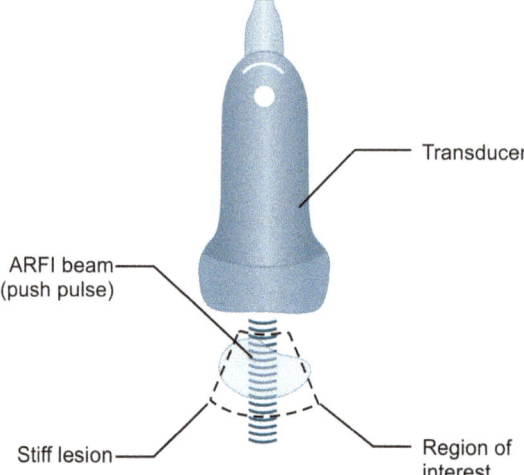

Fig. 6.1: Virtual touch imaging utilizes acoustic push pulses (blue) and detection echo (not shown), sequenced across a user defined region of interest, to generate a displacement map depicting the relative stiffness of tissue.

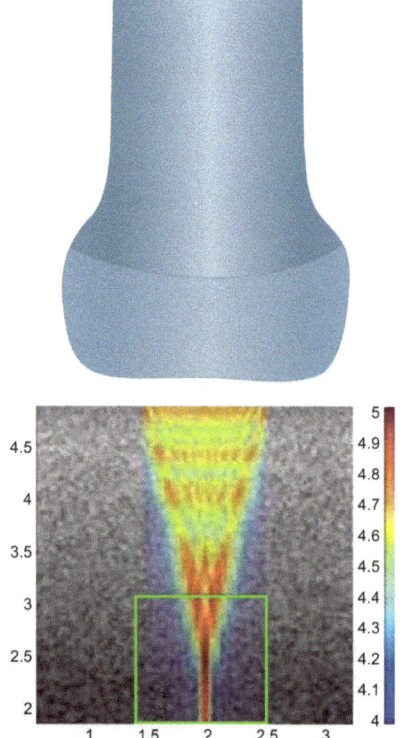

Fig. 6.2: Acoustic radiation force impulse (ARFI) beam with color representation of acoustic intensity: red represents highest intensity, lighter colors represent lower intensity.

Chapter 6: Acoustic Radiation Force Impulse Imaging | 37

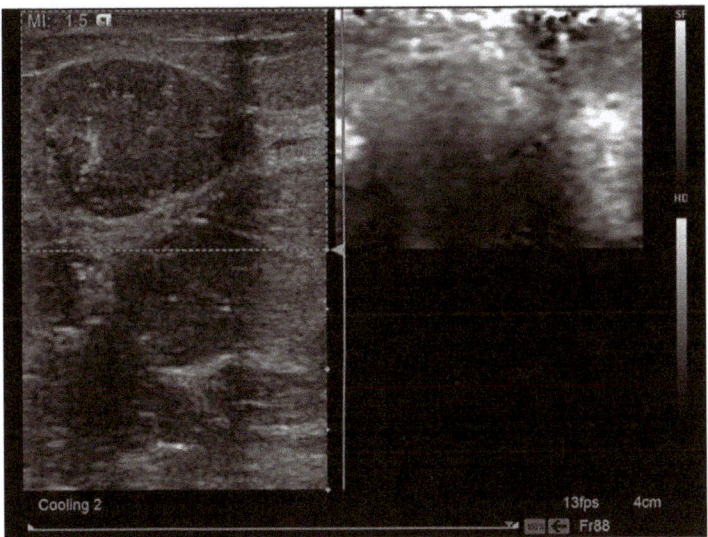

Fig. 6.3: Dual image of B-mode and grayscale VTI image of an oval, slightly hypoechoic, well-defined lesion and presence of calcifications. The lesion appears as dark as the surrounding tissue in the grayscale VTI image. Pathology-proven fibroadenoma.

Virtual Touch Image in Color Map

Virtual touch image in grayscale is illustrated in Figure 6.4.

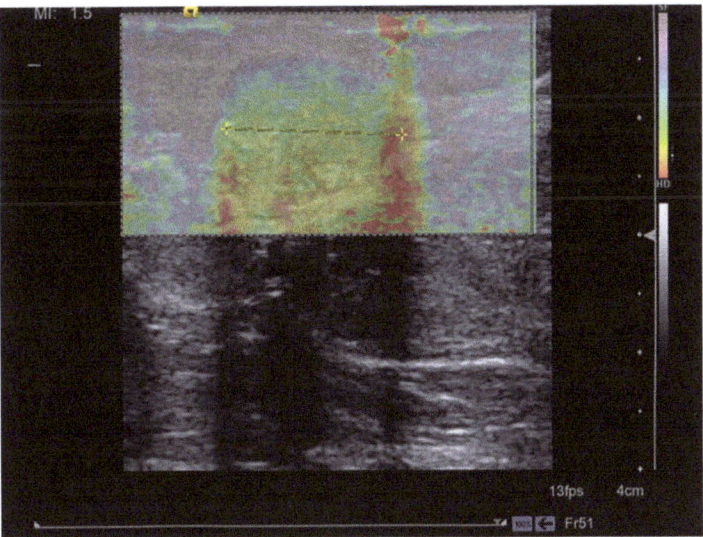

Fig. 6.4: Pathology-proven fibroadenoma (Fig. 6.3) is depicted in VTI color map image as mostly green (soft). The color map besides is indicative of the softness/stiffness of the lesion. Purple and green are indicative of softness, whereas yellow and red are indicative of stiffness.

Qualitative Evaluation of VTI Grayscale Image

Shuang-Ming et al. studied the usefulness of ARFI imaging in the differential diagnosis of benign and malignant liver lesions and described a four-category VTI image evaluation. The categories are the following:
- "Softer" when the lesion appears whiter/brighter than the surrounding breast tissue (Fig. 6.5).

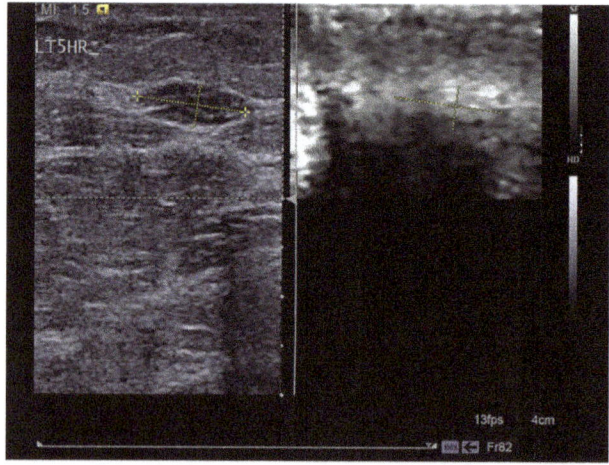

Fig. 6.5: Pathology-proven tubular adenoma. Dual image of B-mode depicting an oval, hypoechoic, well-defined mass and VTI grayscale image with the lesion depicting brighter than the surrounding tissue.

- "Equal stiffness" when the lesion appears with similar brightness to the peripheral breast tissue (Fig. 6.6).

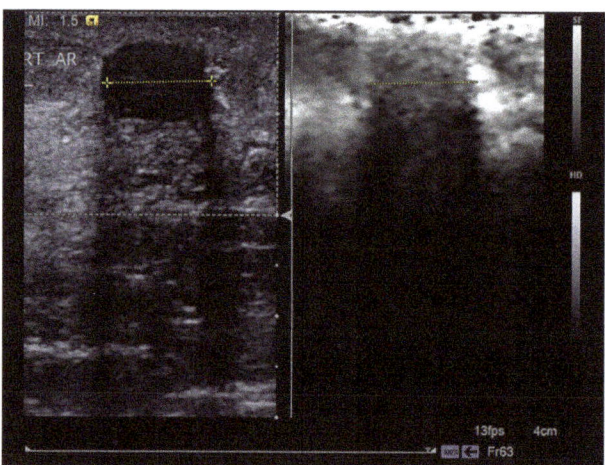

Fig. 6.6: Pathology-proven fibroadenoma with degeneration. The oval, hypoechoic, well-defined, with edge shadowing lesion appears in VTI grayscale image as "equal stiffness" with the surrounding breast tissue.

- "Stiffer" when the lesion is darker (>50%) than the surrounding breast tissue (Fig. 6.7).

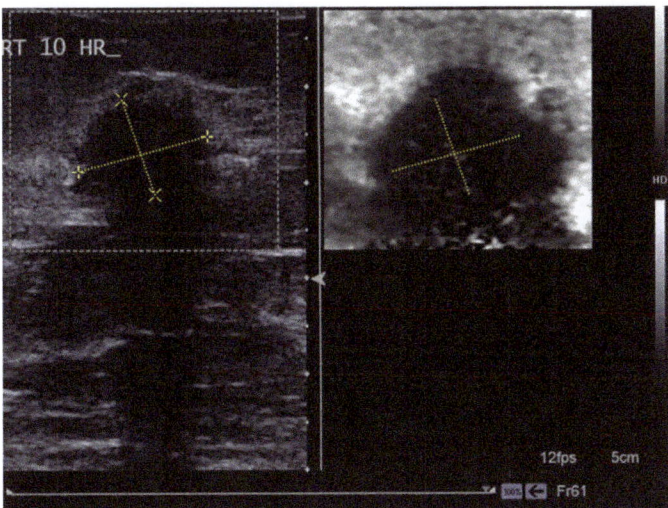

Fig. 6.7: Pathology-proven invasive ductal carcinoma grade III. The ill-defined, marked hypoechoic, with posterior shadowing lesion depicted in B-mode appears darker than the surrounding breast tissue in VTI grayscale image.

- "Cellular sample" when the lesion shows an alternating black and white honeycomb-like distribution (probably caused by separation of tumor cells and multiple fibrous tissues) (Fig. 6.8).

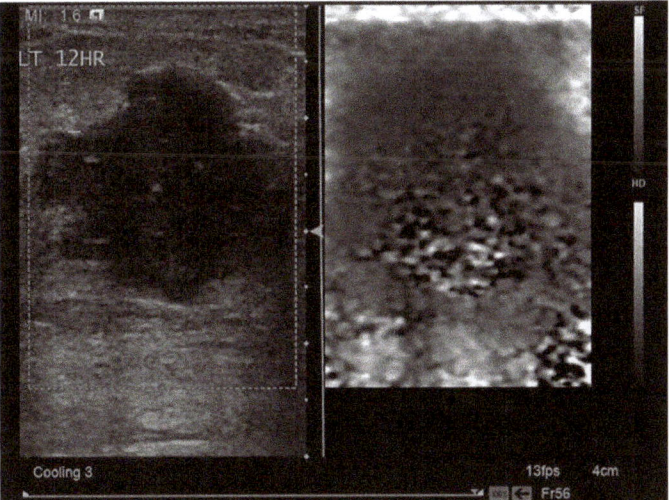

Fig. 6.8: Pathology-proven invasive ductal carcinoma grade III. The ill-defined, marked hypoechoic, with microcalcifications and spiculations mass appears with the typical "cellular sample" in the VTI grayscale image.

Bai M et al. 2015 studied which features are most efficient in the differential diagnosis of solid breast masses with different sizes with ARFI technology and described a four-pattern VTI grayscale image categorization.

According to Bai M et al., the four patterns are the following:
- Pattern 1: VTI grayscale image depicts a bright area corresponding to the lesion in B-mode US (Fig. 6.9).

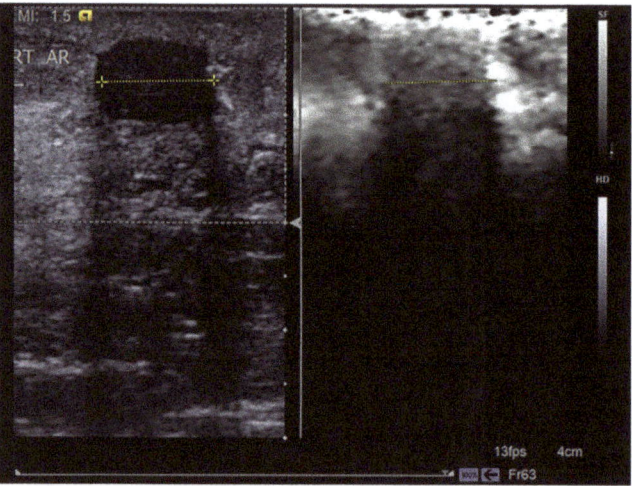

Fig. 6.9: VTI grayscale image depicts a bright area corresponding to the hypoechoic mass in B-mode US.

- Pattern 2: VTI grayscale image depicts no bright or dark areas corresponding to the lesion in B-mode US (Fig. 6.10).

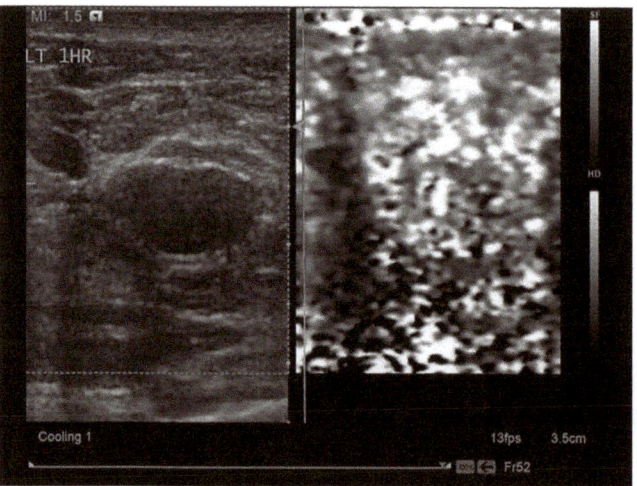

Fig. 6.10: VTI grayscale image depicts no bright or dark areas corresponding to the hypoechoic mass in B-mode US.

- Pattern 3: VTI grayscale image depicts a dark (gray) area corresponding to the lesion in B-mode US (Fig. 6.11).

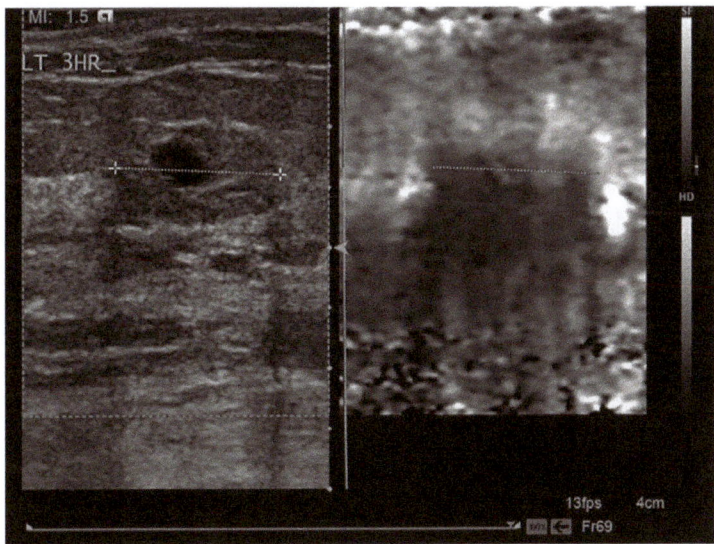

Fig. 6.11: VTI grayscale depicts a dark (gray) area corresponding to the mixed (solid with cystic area) lesion in B-mode US.

- Pattern 4: VTI grayscale image depicts a dark (black) area corresponding to the lesion in B-mode US (Fig. 6.12).

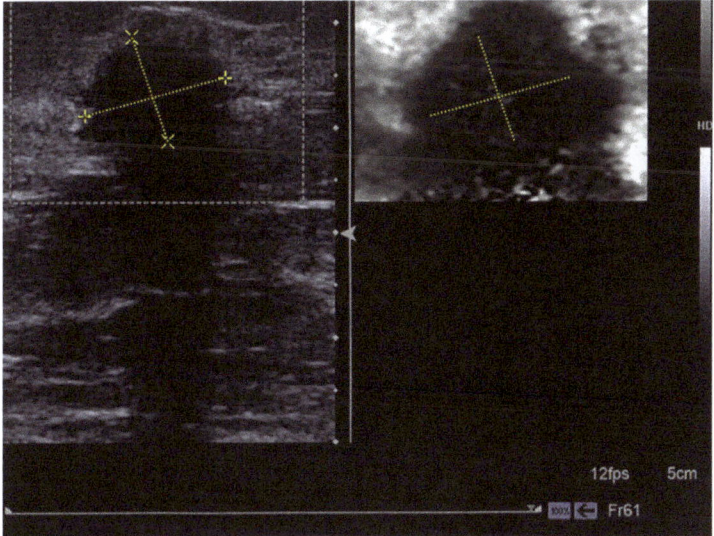

Fig. 6.12: VTI grayscale image depicts a dark (black) area corresponding to the marked hypoechoic mass in B-mode US.

Note that in this book all the clinical cases which are interpreted will be evaluated according to Tian et al. classification.

Evaluation of Color Map VTI Image

Besides to the VTI image, there is a color map according to the hardness is coded as purple, blue, green, yellow, and red which from soft to hard. Green represents the average hardness of tissue elasticity in the US sampling frame. Red and yellow indicate that the hardness of the ROI is greater than the average hardness (Figs. 6.13 and 6.14). Purple and blue indicate that the hardness of the selected area is less than the average hardness (Fig. 6.15).

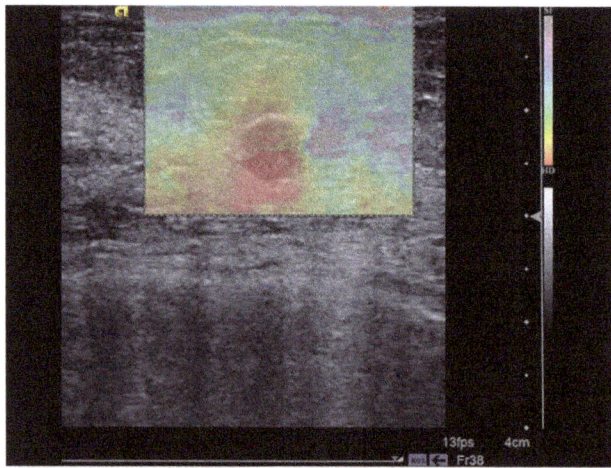

Fig. 6.13: Pathology-proven invasive ductal carcinoma grade III. The ROI appears red.

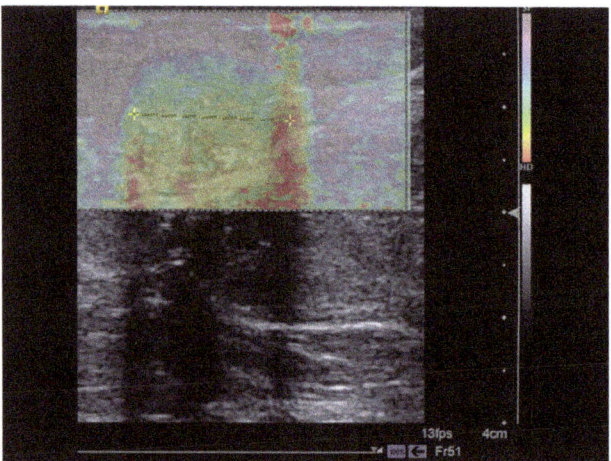

Fig. 6.14: Pathology-proven fibroadenoma is depicted in color map VTI image as mostly yellow but also with green areas.

Chapter 6: Acoustic Radiation Force Impulse Imaging 43

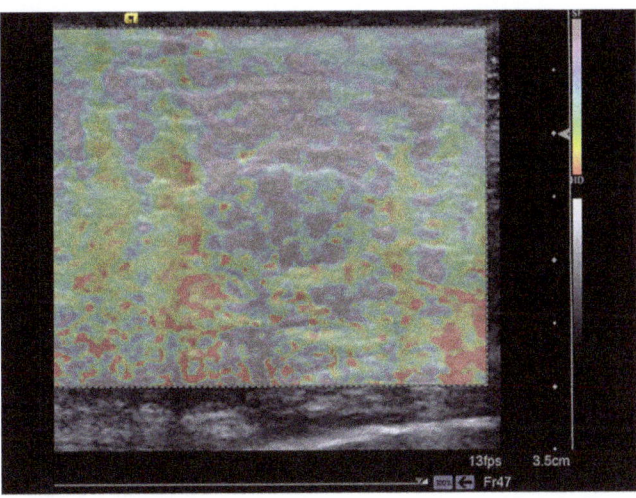

Fig. 6.15: Pathology-proven fibroadenoma is depicted in color map VTI image as mostly purple but also with green and blue areas.

VIRTUAL TOUCH QUANTIFICATION

By combining shear wave velocity measurement with ARFI push pulses, virtual touch quantification (VTQ) measures tissue stiffness directly rather than only relative to surrounding tissues. When an acoustic push pulse displaces the tissue residing in its path, shear waves are generated. These shear waves propagate perpendicular to the push pulse (Fig. 6.16). In tissue, shear

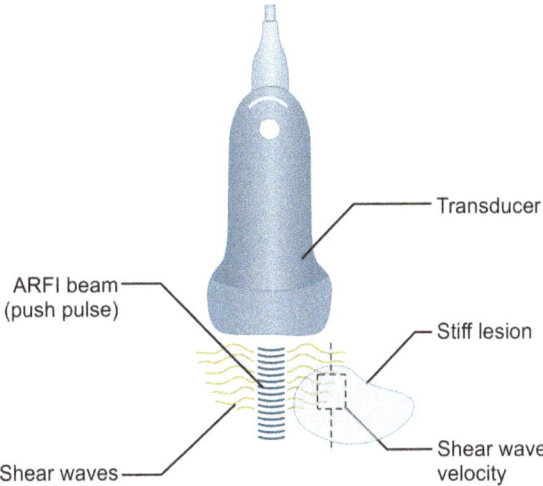

Fig. 6.16: Virtual touch quantification utilizes an acoustic push pulse (blue) to generate shear waves (green) through a user-defined region of interest. Detection pulses are applied in multiple locations and reveal arrival time, allowing quantification of shear wave propagation speed and therefore correlation of tissue stiffness.

waves travel at a velocity of around 1-10 m/sec, which is slow enough to be well sampled by detection beams. There is a close correlation between tissue elasticity and its associated shear wave velocity. By observing the shear wave front arrival at multiple locations and correlating these locations with the arrival time, shear wave speed within the ROI is calculated.

The US transducer both generates the focused ARFI beam and receives echo signal. The ARFI beam is most intense at a selected depth within the tissue. The magnitude of tissue displacement decreases when distance from the ARFI beam increases, and the magnitude in the same spatial location changes over time (Fig. 6.17).

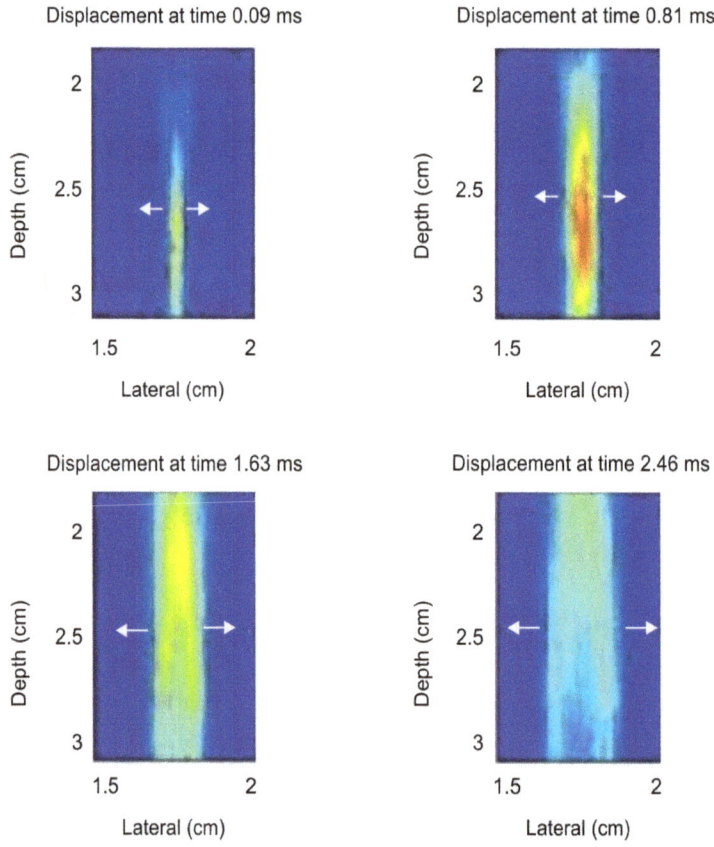

Fig. 6.17: Illustration of tissue displacement information (both its spatial location and magnitude) after ARFI application. The four images show the displacement information at four observation times 0.09, 0.81, 1.63, and 2.63 ms after the cessation of ARFI. The spatial scales in the four images are identical and the arrows in each image indicate that the spatial location of the displaced tissue moves outward perpendicular to the ARFI beam application direction.

The VTQ values (shear wave speed, m/sec) of the lesion are obtained by placing the fixed size ROI on the lesion and subsequently on the adjacent breast tissue in the same depth, where it is possible. The shear waves propagate faster in stiffer tissue (Figs. 6.18 and 6.19).

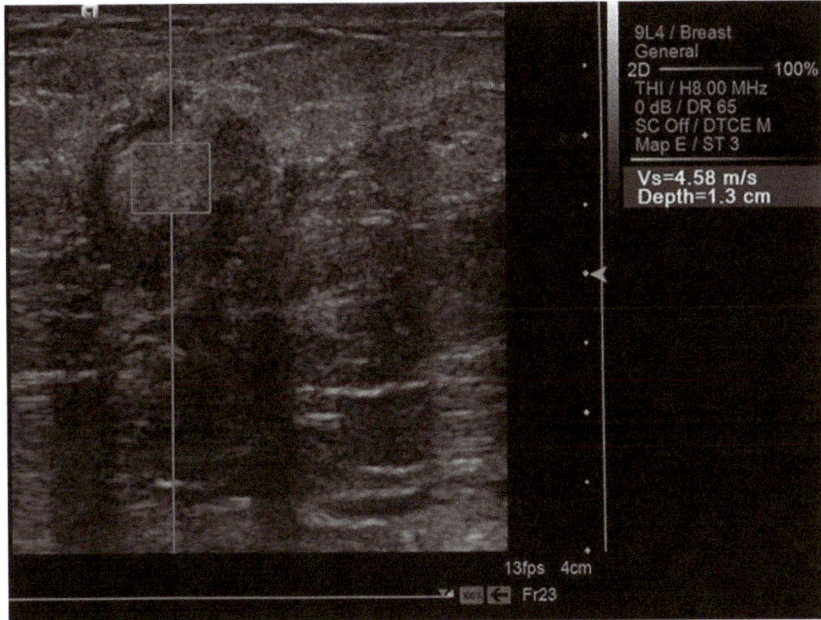

Fig. 6.18: Pathology-proven ductal adenocarcinoma grade III, with foci of ductal carcinoma in situ (DCIS) grade III with microcalcifications. Shear wave velocity inside the lesion is calculated automatically and is equal to 4.58 m/sec.

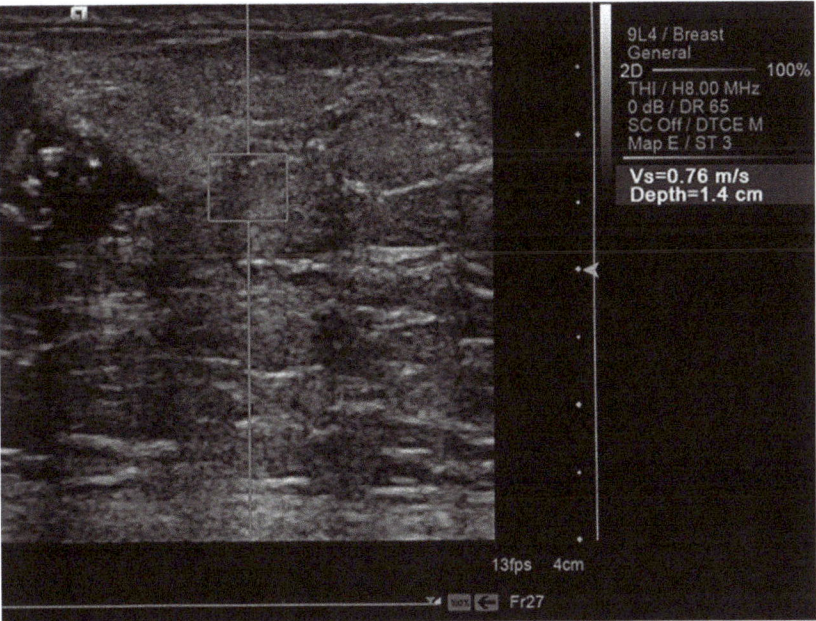

Fig. 6.19: Shear wave velocity in the adjacent breast tissue in the same depth of the case presented in Figure 6.18 is equal to 0.76 m/sec.

Tozaki M et al., studied the combination of elastography and tissue quantification using the ARFI technology for differential diagnosis of breast masses and found that using a shear wave speed cut-off of 3.6 m/sec (38 kPa) a sensitivity of 91% and a specificity of 80.6% were achieved for characterizing breast masses (Figs. 6.20 and 6.21).

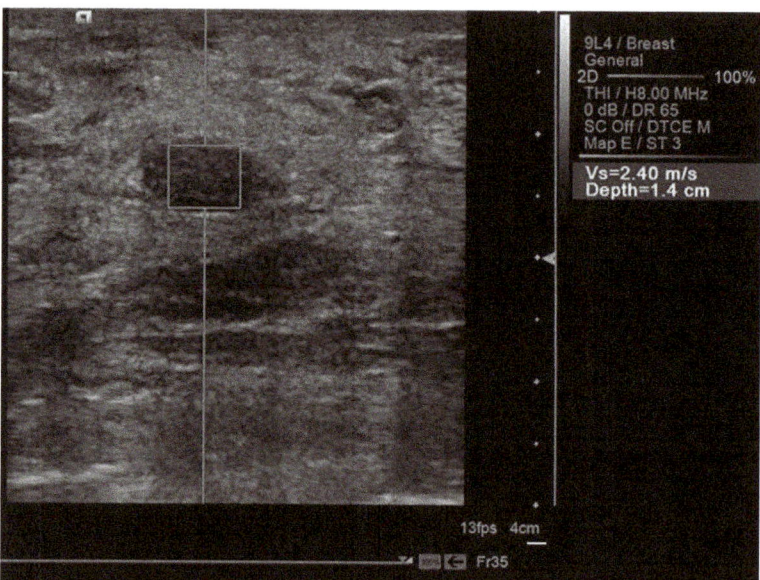

Fig. 6.20: Pathology-proven fibroadenoma. VTQ value inside the lesion is equal to 2.40 m/sec.

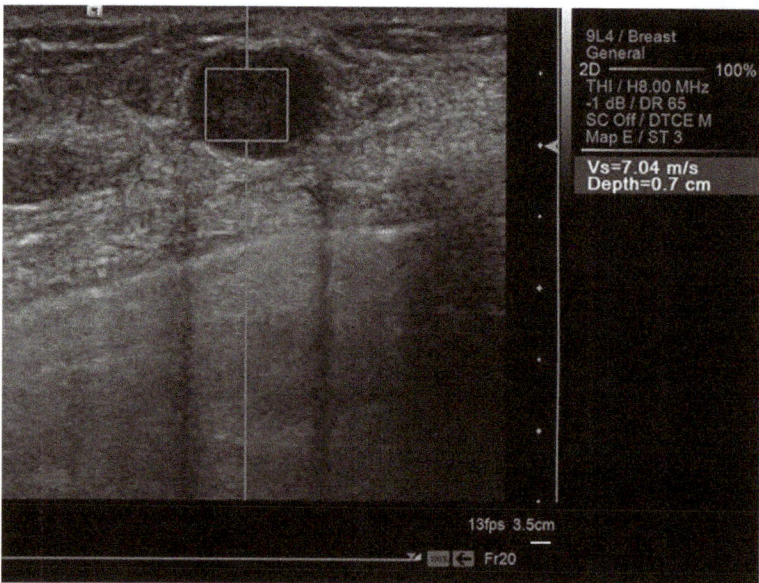

Fig. 6.21: Pathology-proven ductal adenocarcinoma. VTQ value inside the lesion is 7.04 m/sec. Note the benign characteristics of the lesion (well-defined, with edge shadowing).

VIRTUAL TOUCH IQ

Virtual touch IQ (VTIQ) provides the advantage of both quantitative and relative stiffness imaging combined in one display. The user defines a two-dimensional ROI, which represents shear wave velocities at many point locations. The image is formed by a pulse sequence that is comprised of up to 256 acquisition beam lines. For each beam line, the system is instructed to sequentially acquire a noise level estimate, a number of reference vectors, application of ARFI excitation, and then a relative large number of tracking vectors. This sequencing takes place for one single location and gives the estimation of shear wave propagation time for each depth along the beam direction. By taking a similar data acquisition after moving the spatial location of the detection vectors to a location different than the first acquisition, a new line of shear velocity estimates is obtained. This line is in between the detection locations.

To generate an image of shear wave velocities, the above sequencing is repeated for all the lines in a ROI (Fig. 6.22).

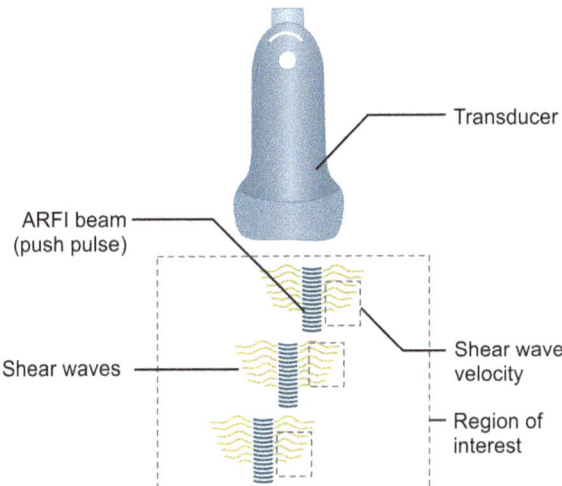

Fig. 6.22: Virtual touch IQ utilizes multiple acoustic push pulses (blue) and multiple detection pulses to provide tissue stiffness quantification throughout a region of interest, rather than in a single location.

The distance between ARFI excitation and detection locations is set as constant when repeating the sequencing across the ROI; therefore, estimating for shear velocity is a function of the travel time and the difference of travel times between detection locations. VTIQ is capable of four discrete shear wave display modes:
1. Velocity
2. Quality
3. Time
4. Displacement

These display modes assist the user in understanding the complex nature of shear waves that may confound image interpretation in the standard shear wave velocity display. The shear wave quality display in particular is useful for interpreting whether the shear wave was of sufficient magnitude with adequate signal-to-noise ratio (SNR) to accurately estimate shear wave velocity in the shear wave velocity display. Shear wave displacement indicates the regions in tissue of low elasticity that may also be associated with higher shear wave velocity. The combination of these display modes provides additional information that when correlated create a better understanding of the shear wave displacement profile.

Notice: VTIQ was not available with our system so, it will not be presented in this edition. May be, a supplement will be included in next publication.

SUGGESTED READING

Bai M, Zhang HP, Xing JF, et al. Acoustic radiation force impulse technology in the differential diagnosis of solid breast masses with different sizes: which features are most efficient? Biomed Res Int. 2015;2015:410560.

Barr RG, Nakashima K, Amy D, et al. WFUMB guidelines and recommendations for clinical use of ultrasound elastography: Part 2: breast. Ultrasound Med Biol. 2015;41 (5):1148-60.

Meng W, Zhang G, Wu C, et al. Preliminary results of acoustic radiation force impulse (ARFI) ultrasound imaging of breast lesions. Ultrasound Med Biol. 2011;37(9):1436-43.

Rosen J, Brown J, De S, et al. Biomechanical properties of abdominal organs in vivo and postmortem under compression loads. J Biomech Eng. 2008;130:021020.

Shuang-Ming T, Ping Z, Ying Q, et al. Usefulness of acoustic radiation force impulse imaging in the differential diagnosis of benign and malignant liver lesions. Acad Radiol. 2011;18(7):810-5.

Tozaki M, Isobe S, Sakamoto M. Combination of elastography and tissue quantification using the acoustic radiation force impulse (ARFI) technology for differential diagnosis of breast masses. Jpn J Radiol. 2012;30(8):659-70.

Wellman P, Howe RH, Dalton E, et al. Breast tissue stiffness in compression is correlated to histological diagnosis. Harvard Biorobotics Laboratory Technical Report, 1999. [online] Available from https://biorobotics. harvard.edu/pubs/1999 /mechprops.pdf. [Accessed March, 2017].

CHAPTER 7
Acoustic Radiation Force Impulse Imaging Examination Protocol

Christina An. Gkali

PATIENT POSITIONING

- The patient lies on her back with her ipsilateral hand raised on the examination bed.
- The medial half of the breast is examined in the supine position.
- The lateral aspect of the breast is examined in supine oblique position (either right or left) with a foam pad positioned under the examined side of the patient.
- The patient is asked to remain and breath calmly.
- A sufficient amount of gel is applied on the skin.
- A linear transducer (4–9 MHz) is positioned perpendicular to the skin.
- A very light compression is applied to the probe.

VIRTUAL TOUCH TISSUE IMAGING EXAMINATION PROTOCOL

- The patient is asked to hold her breath.
- The virtual touch tissue imaging (VTI) option is selected and the region of interest (ROI) encircles the lesion. A button named "Select" is pressed and a black-and-white VTI image is obtained and displayed on a dual screen with the left side showing the B-mode image and the right side showing the elastic image.
- When the button "Select" is pressed twice it gives the sonographer the choice to obtain a color map VTI image. The ROI encircles the lesion and the surrounding tissue and a color map VTI image is obtained in order to compare the stiffness of the lesion with the surrounding tissue according to the color map of the whole selected area, with purple representing soft tissue, green intermediate stiffness tissue and red stiff tissue.

VIRTUAL TOUCH QUANTIFICATION (VTQ) EXAMINATION PROTOCOL

- A very light pressure is applied to the probe.
- The patient is instructed to hold her breath.
- Virtual touch quantification (VTQ) option is selected and the ROI is placed inside the lesion. The shear wave velocity (recorded in m/sec) inside the lesion is calculated automatically. Subsequently, the ROI is placed in the surrounding fat tissue at the same depth of the lesion and the shear wave velocity is calculated automatically.

ACQUISITION TIPS

Acquisition tips have been depicted in Box 7.1.

Box 7.1: Acquisition tips.

1. Surrounding breast tissue must be included in the selected image.
2. No prestress with the probe should be applied (only very light pressure), as the tissue stiffness may be affected (increased).
3. The patient should remain and breath calmly. The operator's touch should be adjusted accordingly.
4. Sometimes, virtual touch quantification (VTQ) value cannot be measured and X.XX m/sec appears (Fig. 7.1). It could be due to operator movements, patient respiration, erroneous region of interest (ROI) positioning (for example into necrotic or cystic portion of a lesion) and finally, due to tissue that is too hard and out of the range of the machine.
5. Not all cancers are stiff (for example, mucinous cancer) and not all benign lesions are soft (Fig. 7.2).

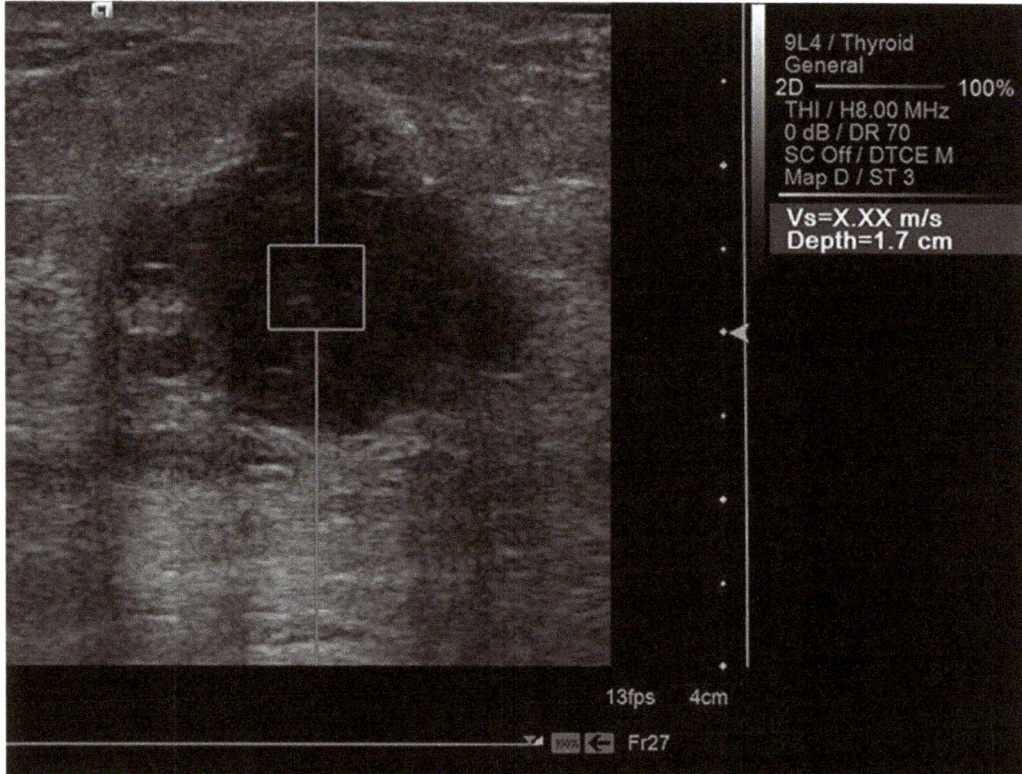

Fig. 7.1: Pathology-proven invasive ductal carcinoma grade III. VTQ value was not feasible to be measured and was recorded as X.XX m/sec.

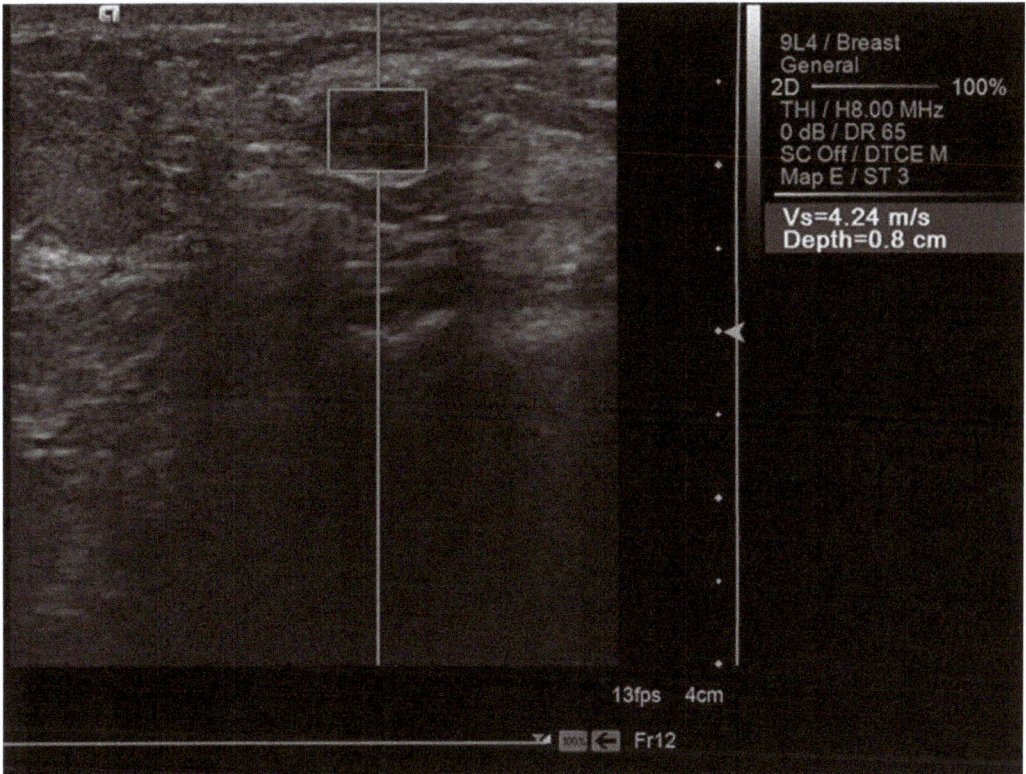

Fig. 7.2: Pathology-proven with high degree of fibrosis. VTQ value was high (4.24 m/sec) affected by microcalcifications.

SUGGESTED READING

Barr RG. Shear wave imaging of the breast: still on the learning curve. J Ultrasound Med. 2012;31:347-50.
Cosgrove D, Piscaglia F, Bamber J, et al. EFSUMB guidelines and recommendations on the clinical use of ultrasound elastography. Part 2: clinical applications. Ultraschall Med. 2013;34:238-53.
Krouskop TA, Wheeler TM, Kallel F, et al. Elastic moduli of breast and prostate tissues under compression. Ultrason Imaging. 1998;20:260-74.
Samani A, Zubovits J, Plewes D. Elastic moduli of normal and pathological human breast tissues: an inversion-technique-based investigation of 169 samples. Phys Med Biol. 2007;52:1565-76.

SECTION 5

SUGGESTED BREAST ULTRASOUND ELASTOGRAPHY REPORTING

CHAPTER 8

Breast Ultrasound Elastography Reporting

Christina An. Gkali

As general guidance, the ultrasound elastography report should be:
- Accurate
- Informative
- Concise
- Easily understood

First of all, the abnormality which is evaluated with elastography should be described and B-mode characteristics, dimensions, precise location within the breast (clock face notation and distance from nipple) should be referred.

Subsequently elastography is performed according to the examination protocols and evaluated as follows.

STRAIN IMAGING

Concerning to strain imaging the information that should be included to a report is the following.

1. Qualitative way of stiffness evaluation:
   - The *elasticity score* has to be evaluated
     - Elasticity score 1–3: Lesion is probably benign
     - Elasticity score 4–5: Probably malignant.
   - The *EI/B ratio* is evaluated (*see* Strain Imaging, Chapter 4):
     - EI/B less than 1: Lesion is probably benign
     - EI/B greater than or equal to 1: Lesion is probably malignant.
2. Semiquantitative way of stiffness evaluation:
   - Strain ratio is calculated automatically (*see* examination protocol, Chapter 4):
     - Strain ratio less than 2.27: Lesion is probably benign
     - Strain ratio greater than 2.27: Lesion is probably malignant.

ACOUSTIC RADIATION FORCE IMPULSE IMAGING

The information that should be included about acoustic radiation force impulse (ARFI) imaging is the following.

Evaluation of the Virtual Touch Tissue Imaging

1. Gray scale:
   - "Softer" or "equal stiffness": Lesion is probably benign
   - "Stiffer" or "cellular sample": Lesion is probably malignant.

2. Color map:
   - *Purple, blue, green*: Lesion is soft
   - *Yellow, red*: Lesion is stiff.

Evaluation of Virtual Touch Tissue Quantification Value

- *Virtual touch tissue quantification (VTQ) value inside the lesion less than 3.6 m/sec*: Lesion is probably benign
- *VTQ value inside the lesion greater than 3.6 m/sec*: Lesion is probably malignant.

BREAK ELASTOGRAPHY REPORT FORM	
Date of Examination	Hospital
	Diagnostic Imaging Departure
Breast Elastography	
Patient details	**Clinical presentation**
Name:	Palpable
Age:	Nodularity
History (family or previous):	Pain
	Mammographic finding
Strain imaging	**Acoustic radiation force impulse (ARFI) imaging**
Elasticity score:	Virtual touch tissue imaging (VTI)
1–3	**Gray scale:**
4–5	Softer
El/B ratio:	Equal stiffness
<1	Stiffer
≥1	Cellular sample
Strain ratio:	Color map:
<2.27	Purple, blue, green
>2.27	Yellow-red
	Virtual touch tissue quantification (VTQ) value:
	<3.6 m/sec
Comments/report	Sonographer/signature

SUGGESTED READING

Barr RG. Real-time ultrasound elasticity of the breast: initial clinical results. Ultrasound Q. 2010;26:61-6.

Fischer T, Peisker U, Fiedor S, et al. Significant differentiation of focal breast lesions: raw data-based calculation of strain ratio. Ultraschall Med. 2012;33:372-9.

Itoh A, Ueno E, Tohno E, et al. Breast disease: clinical application of US elastography for diagnosis. Radiology. 2006;239:341-50.

Shuang-Ming T, Ping Z, Ying Q, et al. Usefulness of acoustic radiation force impulse imaging in the differential diagnosis of benign and malignant liver lesions. Acad Radiol. 2011;18(7):810-5.

Tozaki M, Isobe S, Sakamoto M. Combination of elastography and tissue quantification using the acoustic radiation force impulse (ARFI) technology for differential diagnosis of breast masses. Jpn J Radiol. 2012;30(8):659-70.

SECTION 6

INTERPRETATION OF BENIGN AND MALIGNANT BREAST LESIONS

CHAPTER 9
Interpretation of Benign Breast Lesions

Christina An. Gkali

CASE 1: A 52-year-old woman referred for annual evaluation and underwent B-mode ultrasound and strain ultrasound elastography.

Physical examination: No palpable mass.

B-mode ultrasound findings have been shown in Figure 9.1.

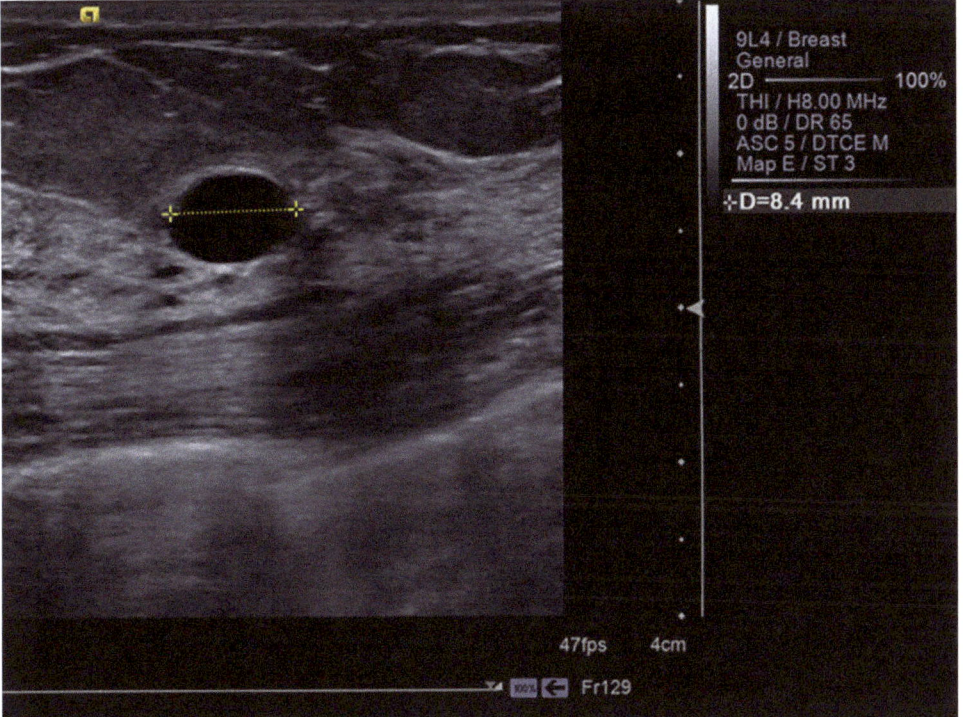

Fig. 9.1: Multiple echo-free, thin-walled, noncomplicated cysts, with maximum diameter 8.4 mm.

Grayscale strain elastography findings have been shown in Figure 9.2.

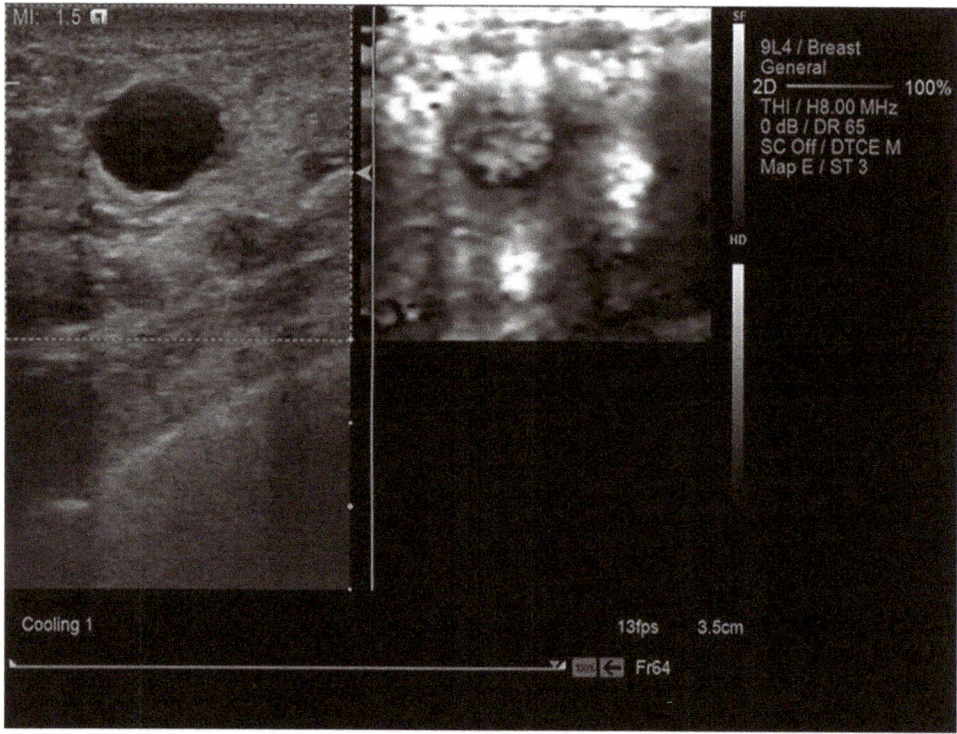

Fig. 9.2: Cysts appear with a typical bull's eye sign (smaller size, white center, black peripheral circle) in the grayscale elastogram (Siemens equipment).

CASE 2: A 20-year-old girl referred for evaluation of a palpable, painful mass of her right breast.

Physical examination: Palpable mass, approximately 2 cm with associated localized breast edema, erythema, warmth, and pain.

B-mode ultrasound findings have been shown in Figure 9.3.

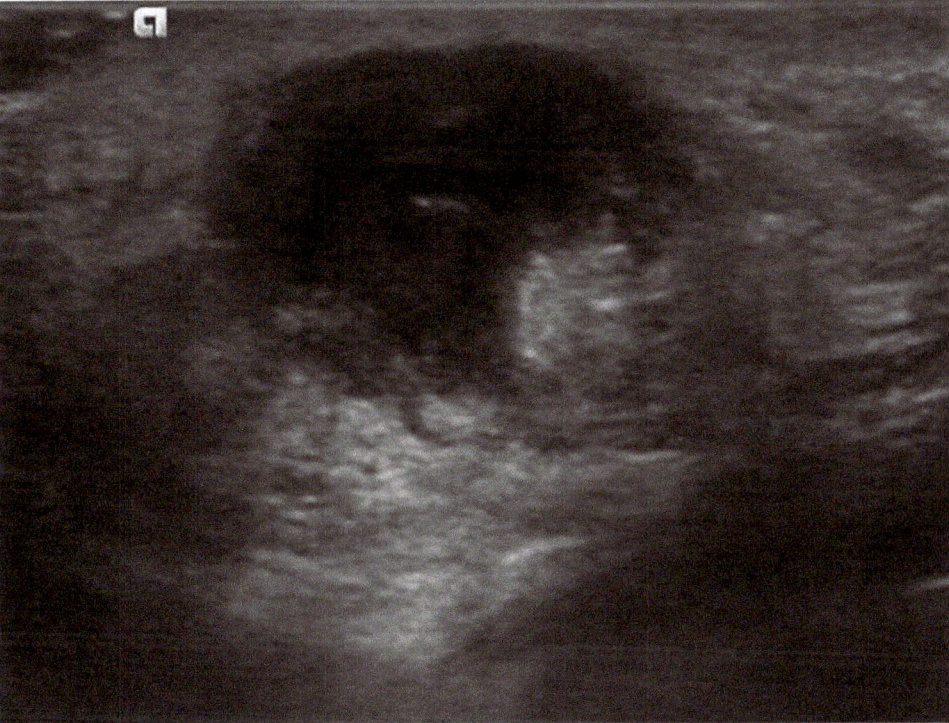

Fig. 9.3: B-mode ultrasound revealed a 2 cm in maximum diameter, mixed mass (anechoic with internal echoes), with irregular margins, posterior enhancement and no internal septae.

Color Doppler findings have been shown in Figure 9.4.

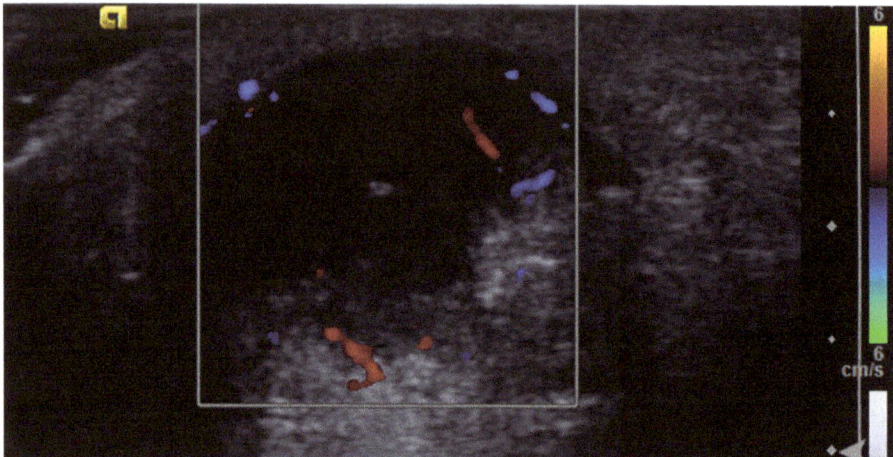

Fig. 9.4: Color Doppler revealed increased vascularity along the rim of the lesion. The ultrasound findings in combination with clinical examination were suggestive of an abscess. The girl underwent drainage of the abscess.

Elasticity score has been shown in Figure 9.5.

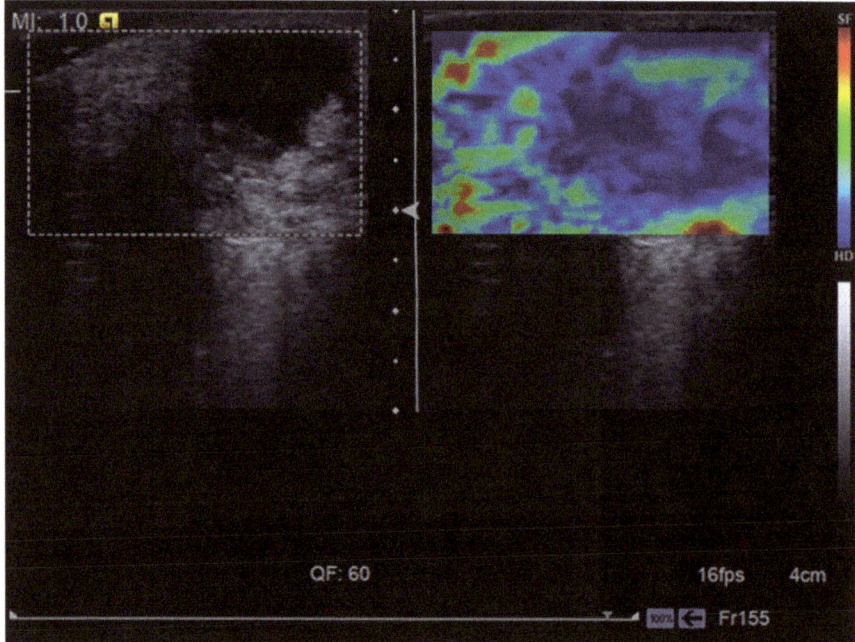

Fig. 9.5: Elasticity score = 3 (the peripheral portion of the lesion is deformable with stiff tissue in the center: blue in the center and green peripherally).

Strain ratio evaluation has been shown in Figure 9.6.

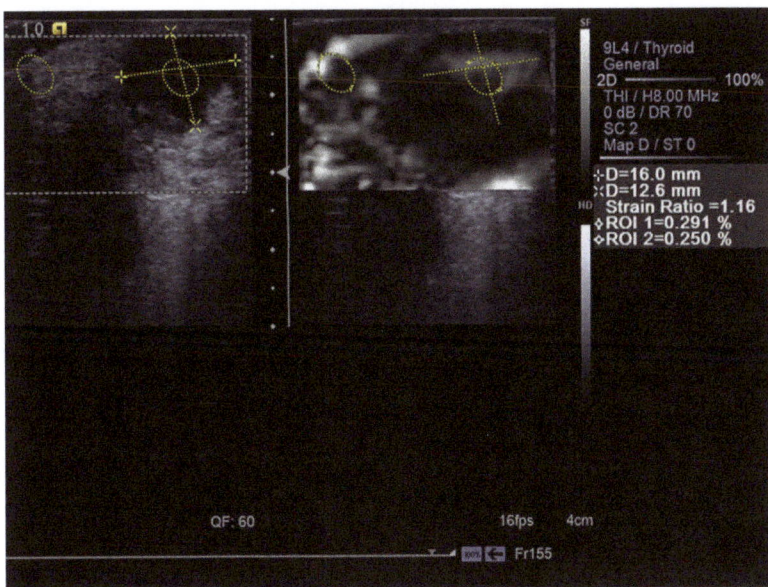

Fig. 9.6: Strain ratio was equal to 1.16.

Virtual touch quantification (VTQ) value estimation inside the lesion has been shown in Figure 9.7.

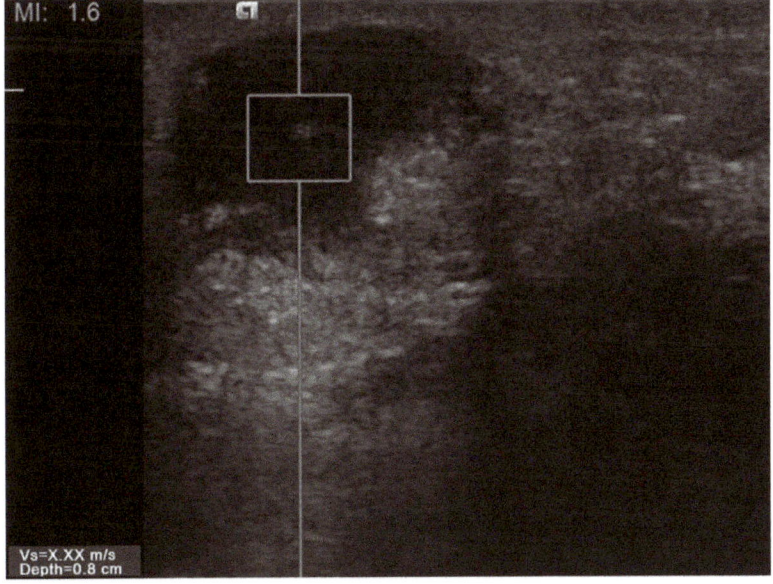

Fig. 9.7: VTQ value was impossible to be calculated and was displayed as X.XX m/sec.

Pathology result has been shown in Figure 9.8.

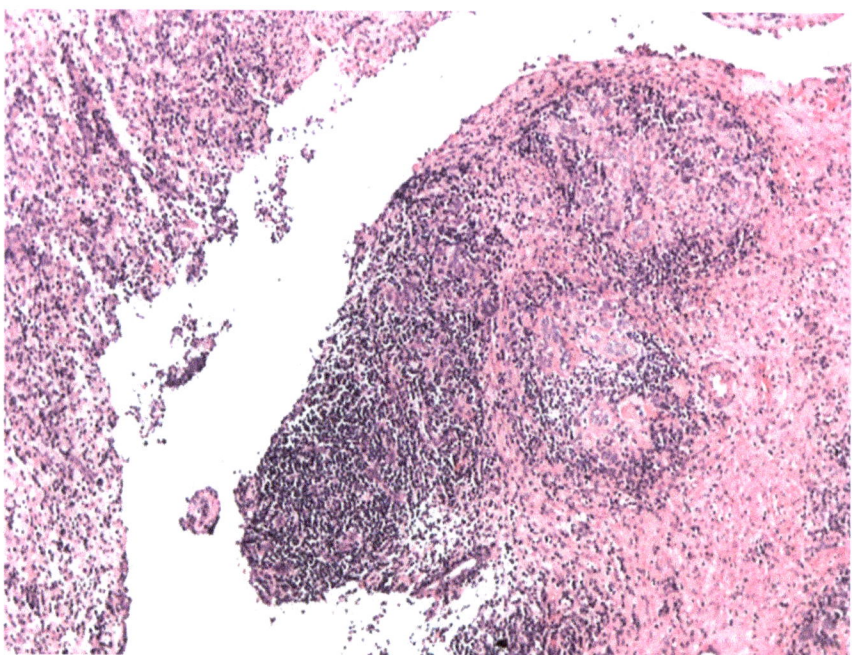

Fig. 9.8: Breast tissue is displaced by chronic active inflammation with lymphocytes, plasma cells and neutrophils.

CONCLUSION

Elastography and pathology results are in concordance.

Notes: Abscesses because of their heterogeneity in their composition may result in a signal that is not accurately identified and this is why VTQ value inside the lesion was impossible to be evaluated and demonstrated as X.XX m/sec.

CASE 3: A 42-year-old woman referred for further evaluation of a mass depicted in screening digital mammography (DM).

Physical examination: Retroareolar, palpable, painless mass of right breast.
B-mode ultrasound findings have been shown in Figure 9.9.

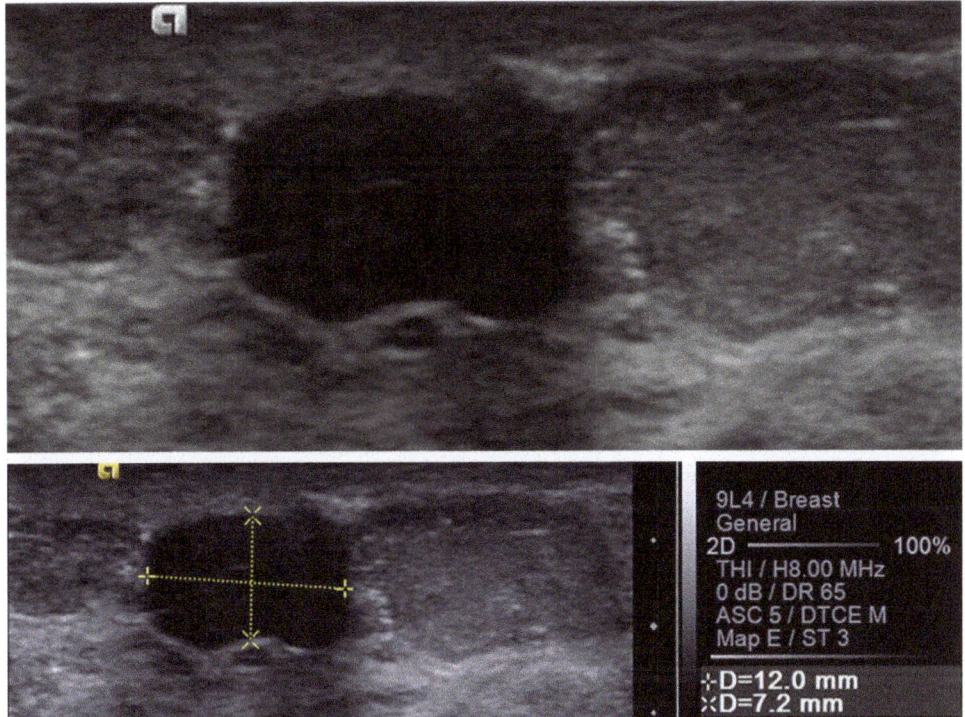

Fig. 9.9: B-mode ultrasound revealed a hypoechoic, well-defined, encapsulated mass, measured 1.2 cm in maximum diameter.

Color Doppler imaging has been shown in Figure 9.10.

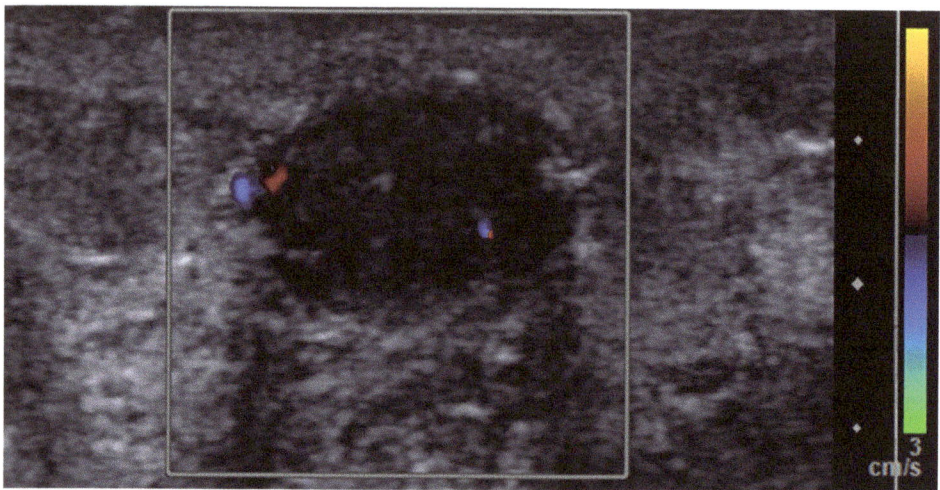

Fig. 9.10: Color Doppler revealed low internal vascularity.

Elasticity score has been shown in Figure 9.11.

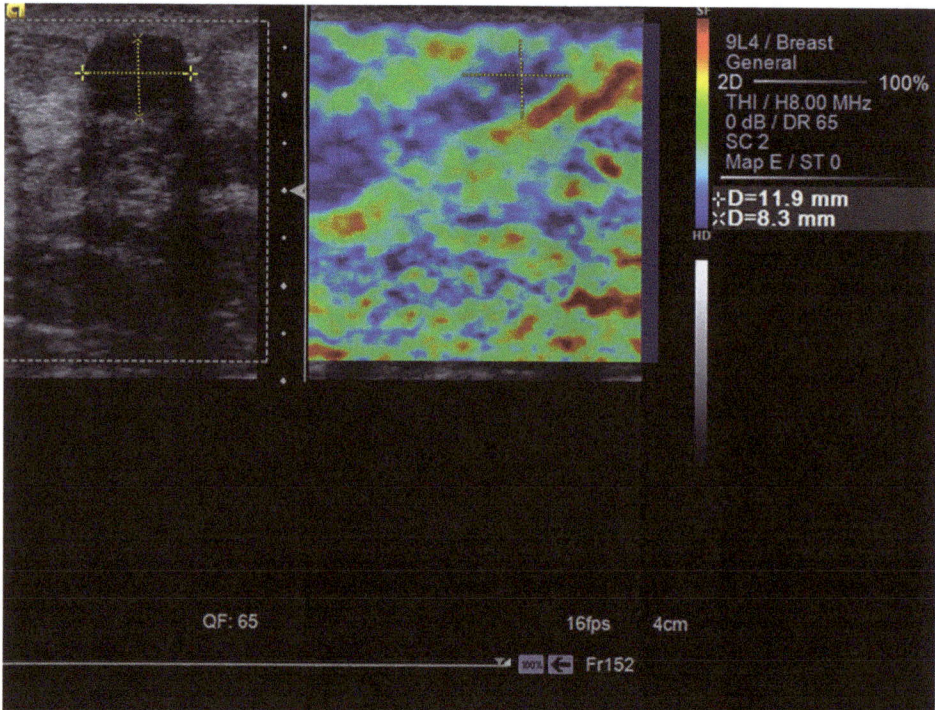

Fig. 9.11: Elasticity score: 3.

Calculation of strain ratio has been shown in Figure 9.12.

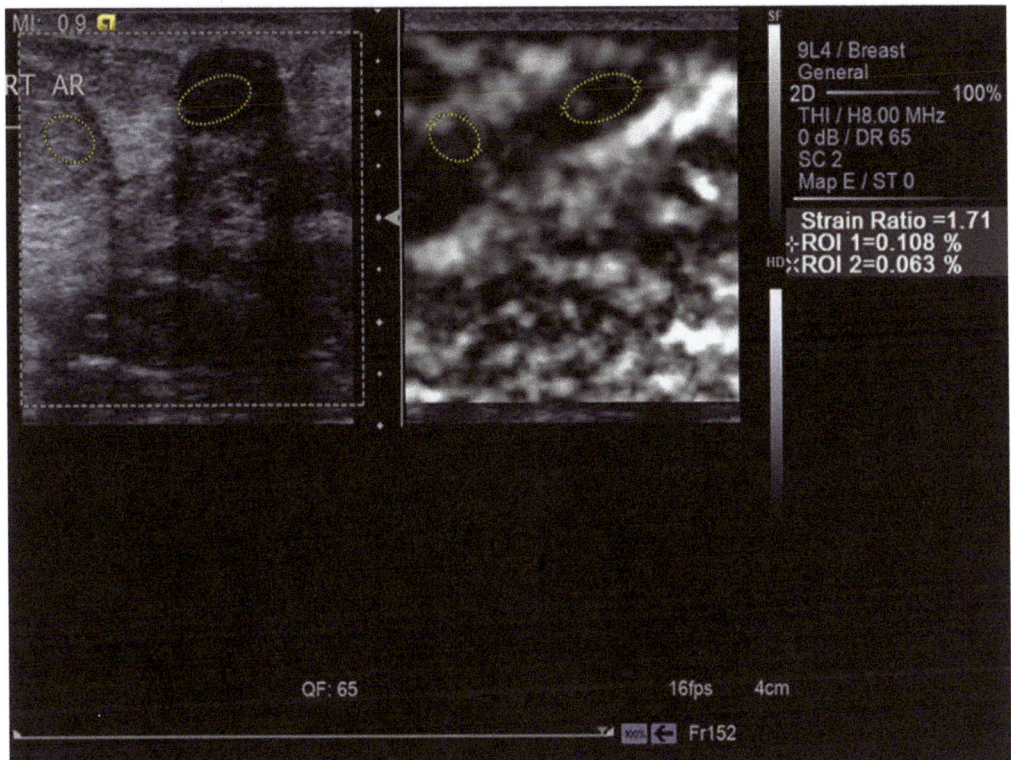

Fig. 9.12: Strain ratio was equal to 1.71.

Grayscale virtual touch imaging (VTI) has been shown in Figure 9.13.

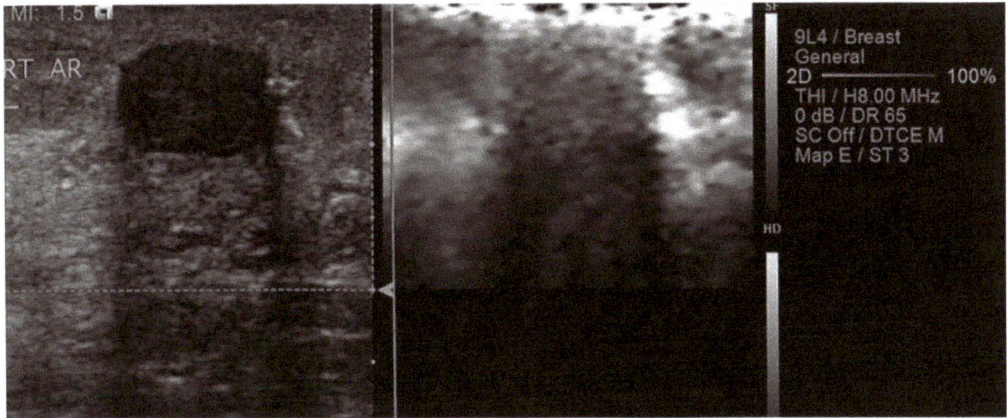

Fig. 9.13: Grayscale VTI image of the lesion is of equal stiffness compared to the surrounding tissue.

Color map VTI imaging has been shown in Figure 9.14.

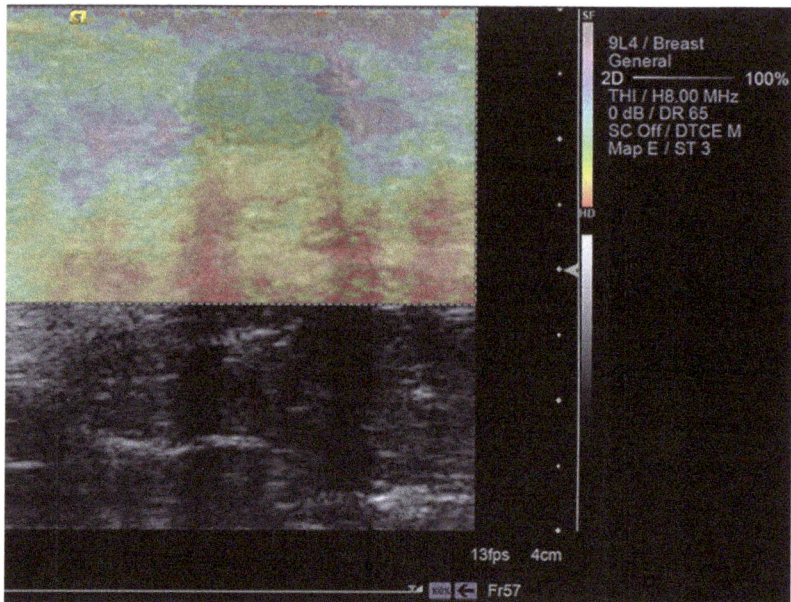

Fig. 9.14: VTI image depicted a green-purple lesion.

Virtual touch quantification value estimation inside the lesion has been shown in Figure 9.15.

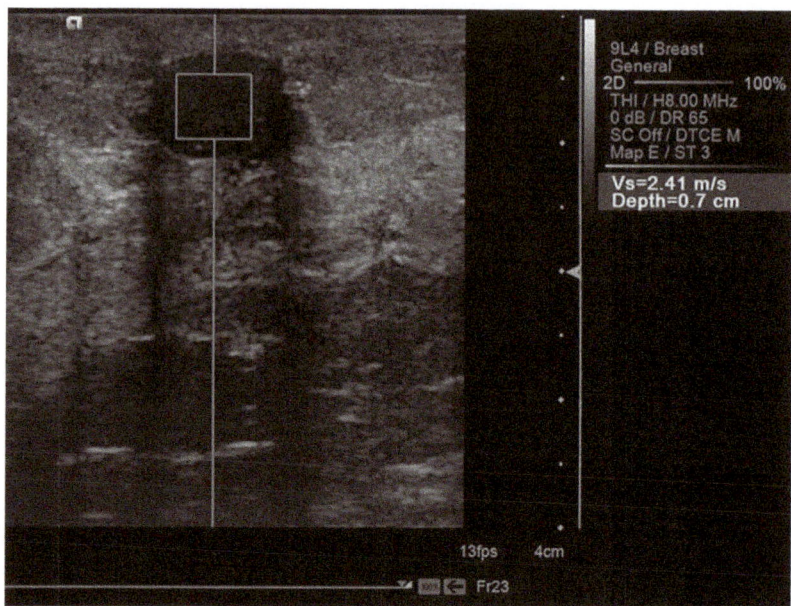

Fig. 9.15: VTQ value inside the lesion was estimated 2.41 m/sec.

Virtual touch quantification value in the surrounding tissue has been shown in Figure 9.16.

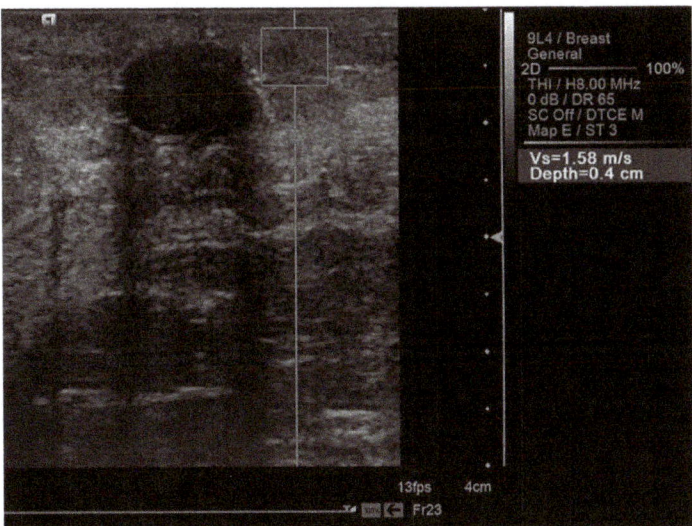

Fig. 9.16: VTQ value in the surrounding tissue is equal to 1.58 m/sec.

Pathology result has been shown in Figure 9.17.

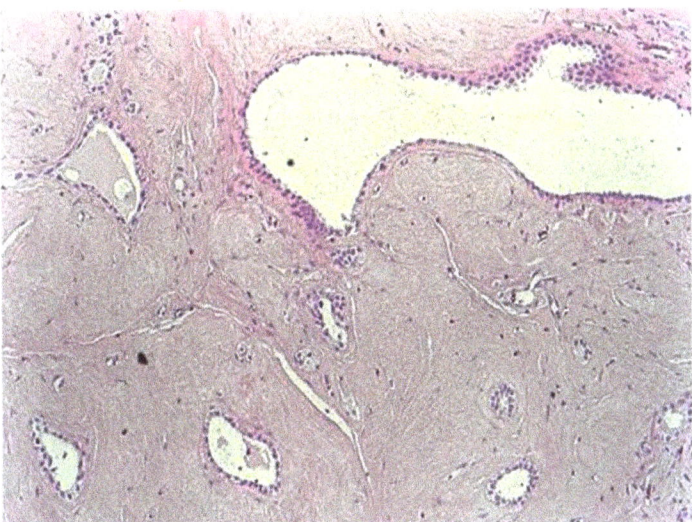

Fig. 9.17: Pathology result was fibroadenoma. Dilated or compressed ducts surrounded by hypocellular stroma.

CONCLUSION

Elastography results were suggestive of benignity and in concordance with pathology result.

CASE 4: A 55-year-old woman.

Physical examination revealed a palpable, painless mass at 3 o' clock of her left breast. *B-mode ultrasound findings* have been shown in Figures 9.18A and B.

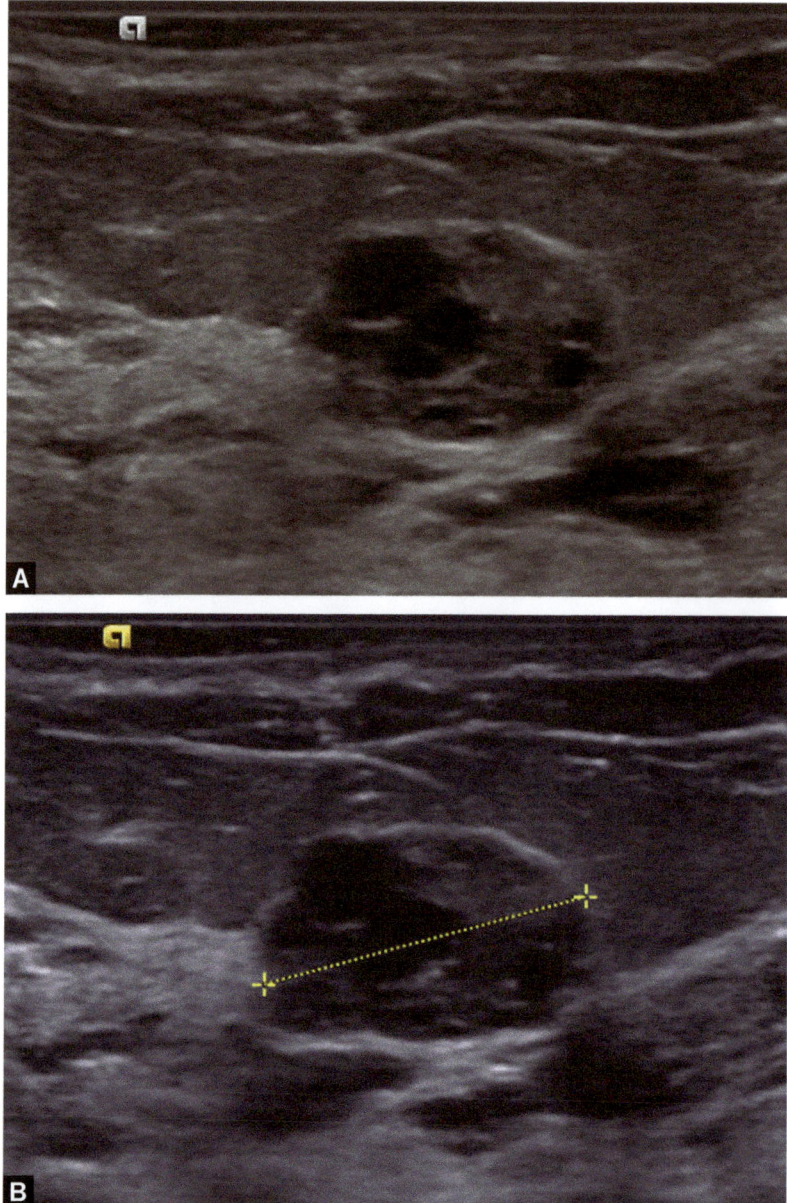

Figs. 9.18A and B: B-mode ultrasound revealed an oval, well-circumscribed, encapsulated, mixed mass (solid mass with cystic parts), measured 1.5 cm in maximum diameter.

Chapter 9: Interpretation of Benign Breast Lesions 73

Color Doppler imaging has been shown in Figure 9.19.

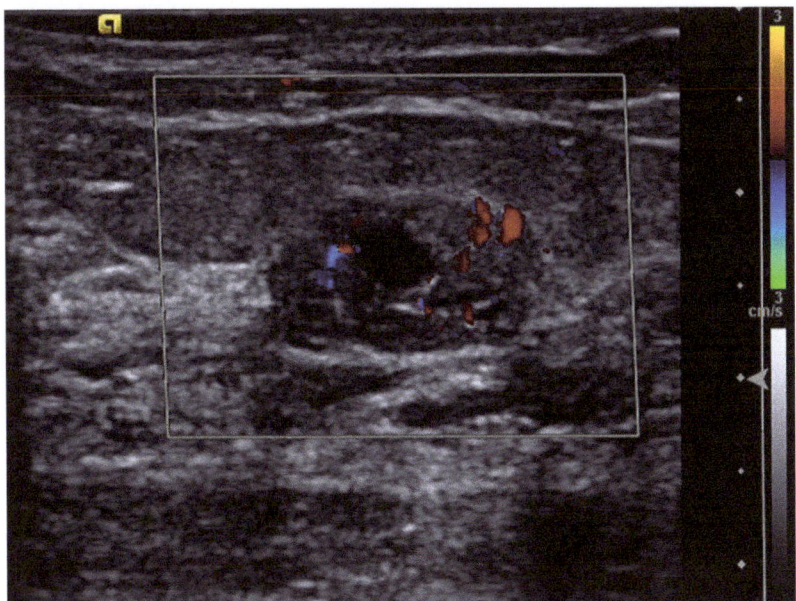

Fig. 9.19: Color Doppler revealed low vascularity in the solid part of the lesion.

Calculation of strain ratio has been shown in Figure 9.20.

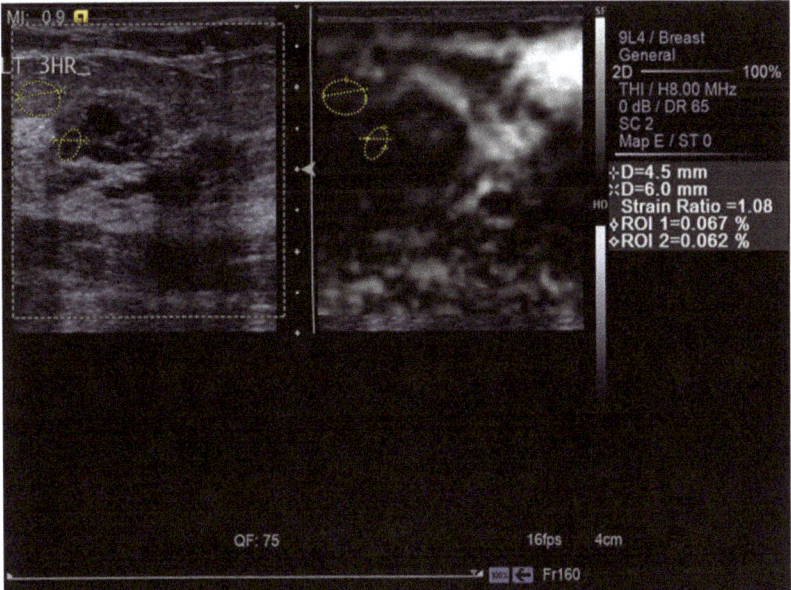

Fig. 9.20: Strain ratio was estimated 1.08.

Notice that the region of interest (ROI) of the lesion encircles only the solid part of the lesion (not the cystic).

Grayscale VTI imaging has been shown in Figure 9.21.

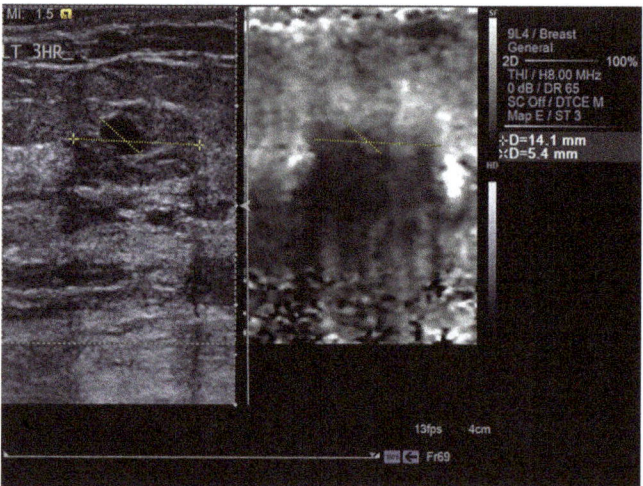

Fig. 9.21: VTI grayscale image revealed a lesion of same darkness with surrounding tissue.

Notice the typical "bull's eye" appearance of the cystic part of the lesion.

Color map VTI imaging has been shown in Figure 9.22.

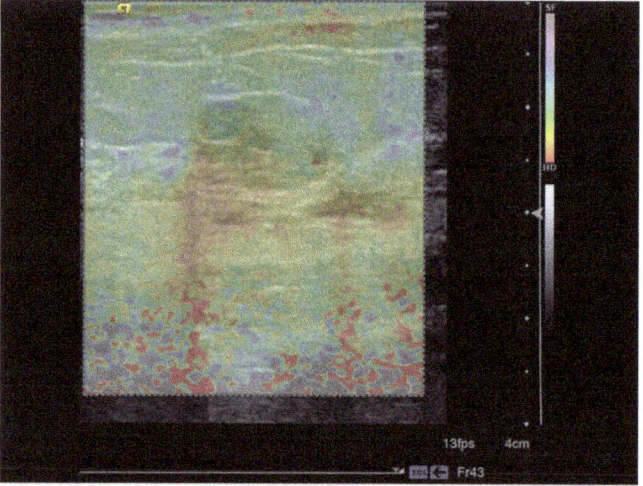

Fig. 9.22: VTI color map image revealed a green (= soft) lesion.

VTQ value estimation inside the lesion has been shown in Figure 9.23.

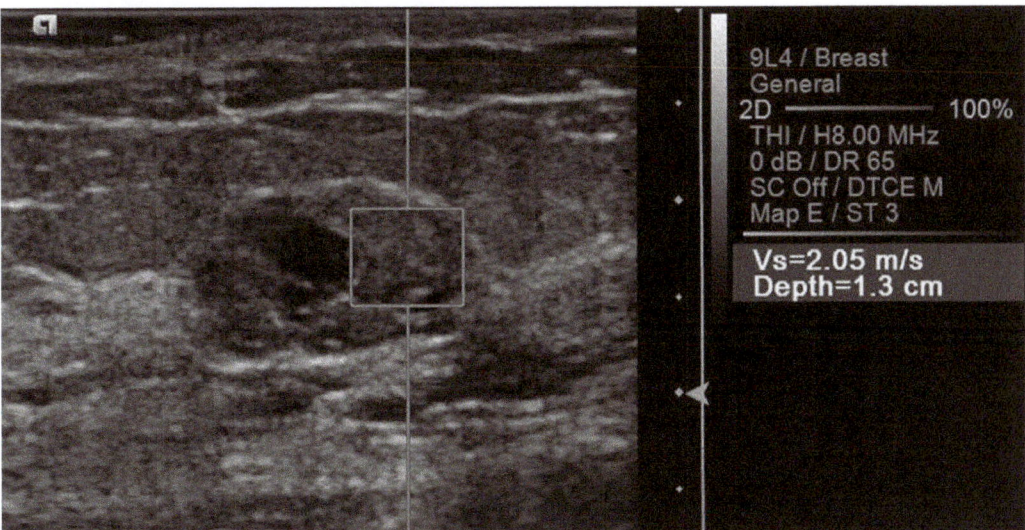

Fig. 9.23: VTQ value inside the lesion was estimated 2.05 m/sec.

Notice that the ROI is placed inside the solid part of the lesion.
VTQ value estimation in the adjacent tissue has been shown in Figure 9.24.

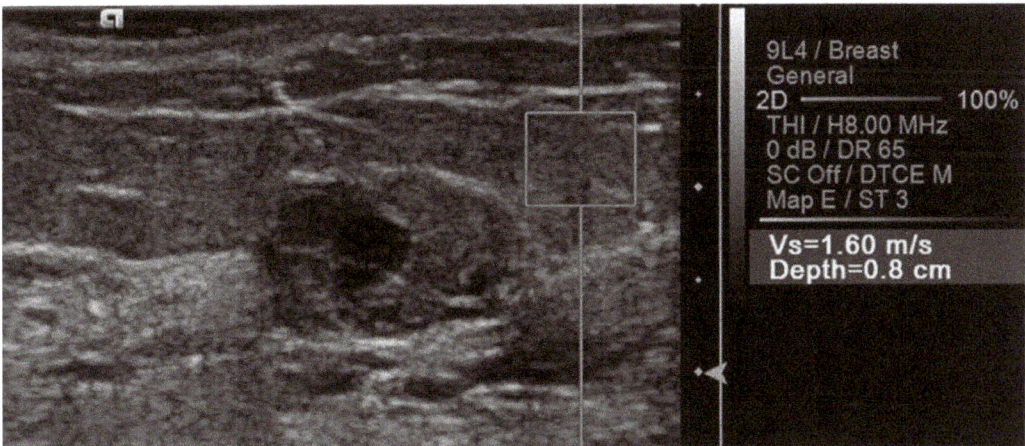

Fig. 9.24: VTQ value in the surrounding tissue (same depth) was 1.60 m/sec.

Pathology result has been shown in Figure 9.25.

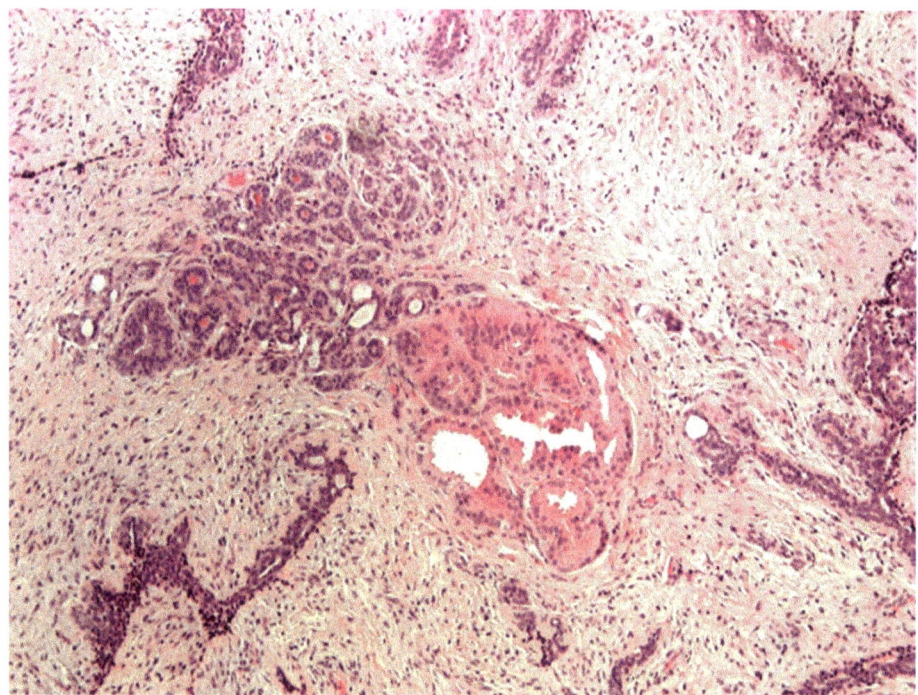

Fig. 9.25: Pathology result was complex fibroadenoma with foci of apocrine metaplasia.

CONCLUSION

The pathology result was in concordance with elastography findings, which were suggestive of a probably benign lesion.

It is important to mention that in mixed masses the ROI (strain ratio calculation, VTQ value estimation of the lesion) must be placed inside the solid part of the lesion.

Chapter 9: Interpretation of Benign Breast Lesions

CASE 5: A 48-year-old woman underwent screening mammography.

Mammographic findings have been shown in Figure 9.26.

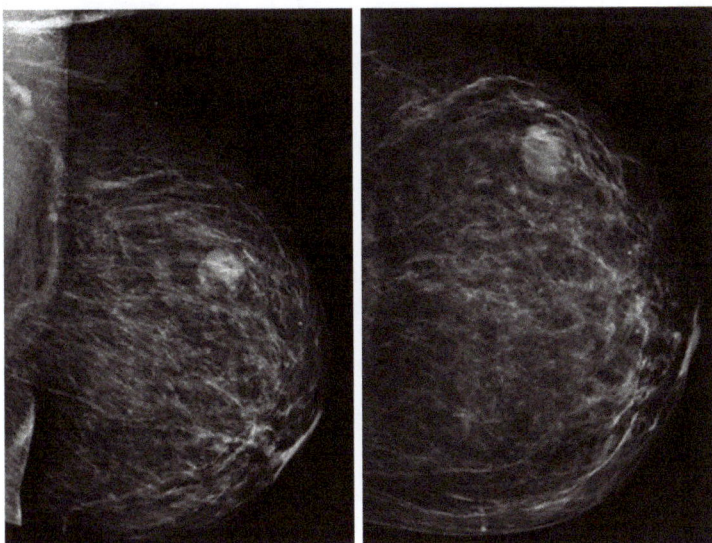

Fig. 9.26: Left breast, craniocaudal (CC) and mediolateral oblique (MLO) views revealed a radiolucent and radiopaque combined lesion.

B-mode ultrasound findings have been shown in Figure 9.27.

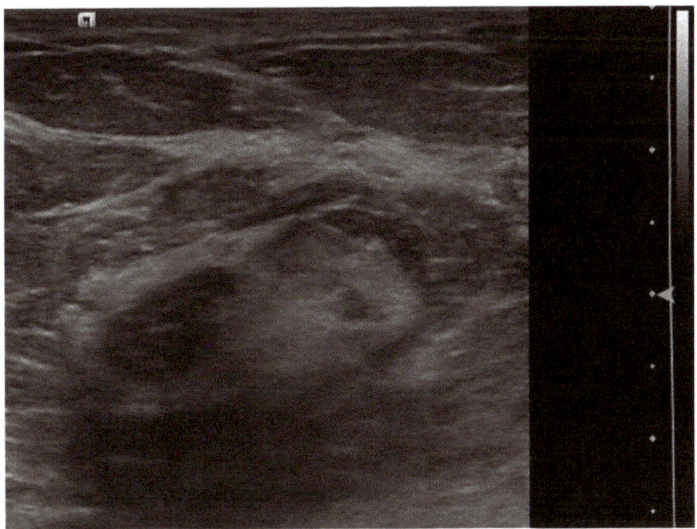

Fig. 9.27: B-mode ultrasound revealed an oval, mixed with combination of hypoechoic and hyperechoic parts.

Color Doppler imaging has been shown in Figure 9.28.

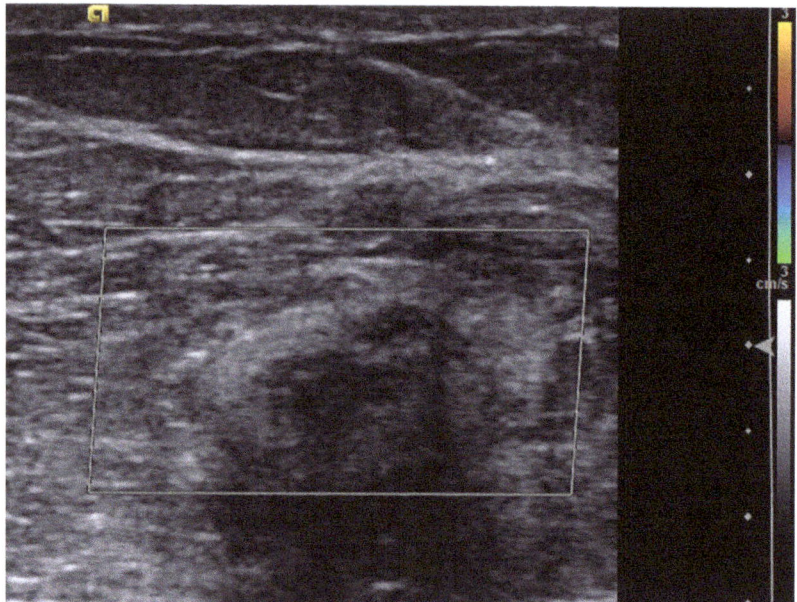

Fig. 9.28: No internal vascularity.

Elasticity score has been shown in Figure 9.29.

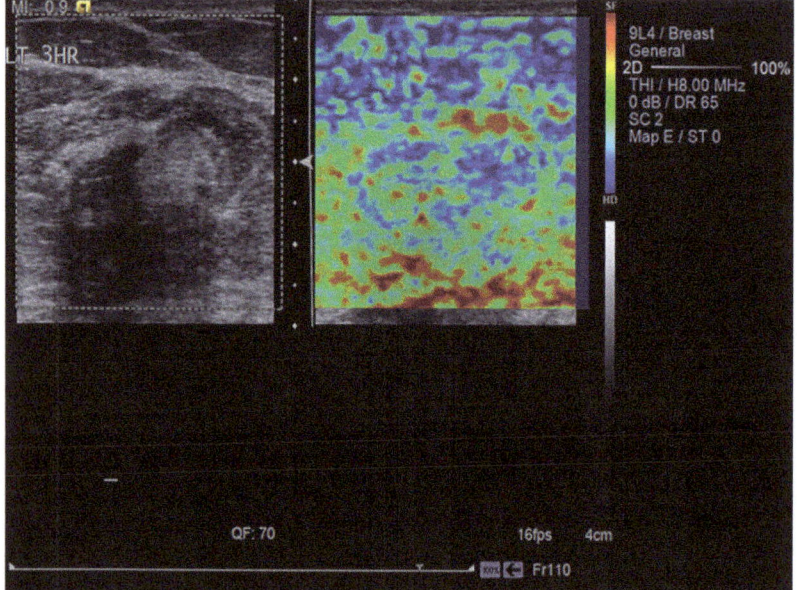

Fig. 9.29: Elasticity score: 2 (soft with stiff areas).

Color map VTI imaging has been shown in Figure 9.30.

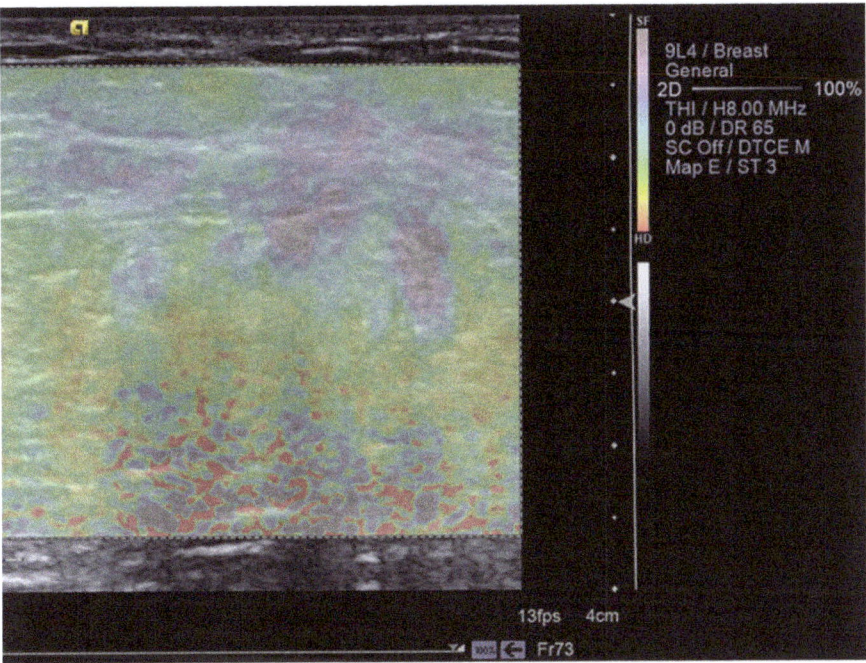

Fig. 9.30: VTI color map imaging revealed a purple-blue-green lesion (= soft).

VTQ value estimation inside the lesion has been shown in Figure 9.31.

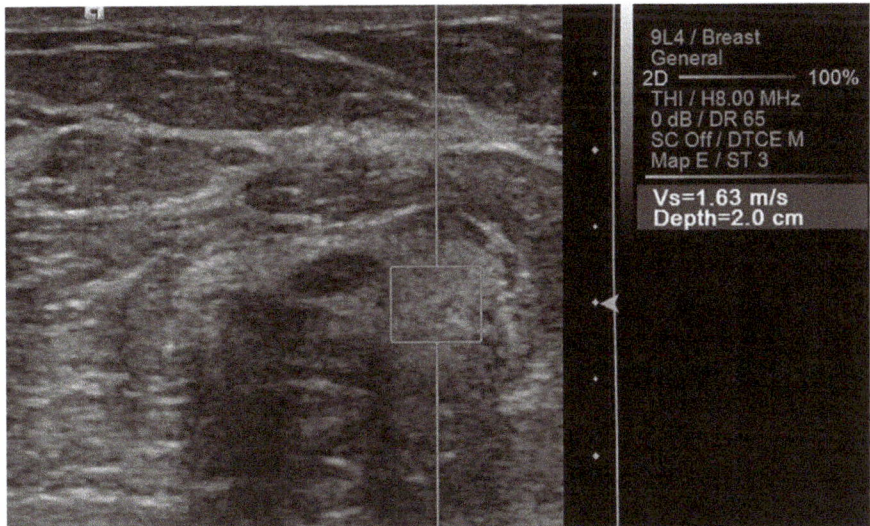

Fig. 9.31: VTQ value inside the lesion was equal to 1.63 m/sec.

Pathology result has been shown in Figure 9.32.

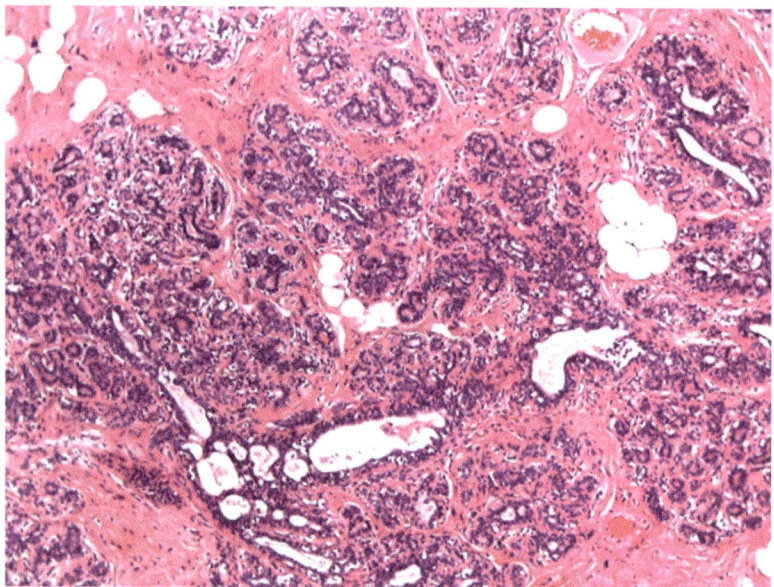

Fig. 9.32: Adenosis—increased number of glandular component.

CONCLUSION

Elastographic findings were suggestive of a probably benign lesion and in concordance with pathology results.

Chapter 9: Interpretation of Benign Breast Lesions | 81

CASE 6: A 35-year-old woman referred for further evaluation of a palpable mass of left breast.

Physical examination: Palpable, painless mass, approximately 3 cm of the left breast.
Digital mammography findings have been shown in Figure 9.33.

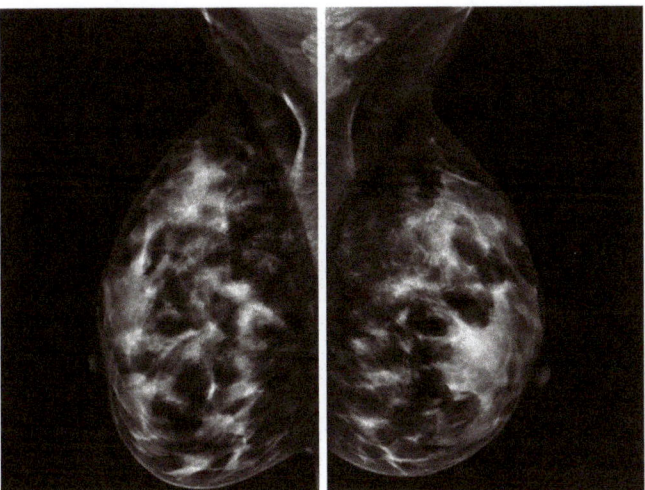

Fig. 9.33: Right and left profile digital mammography (DM) images evaluated as the American College of Radiology (ACR) 3 breast density and breast imaging-reporting and data system (BI-RADS) 0 classification. Additional imaging evaluation was necessary.

B-mode ultrasound findings have been shown in Figure 9.34.

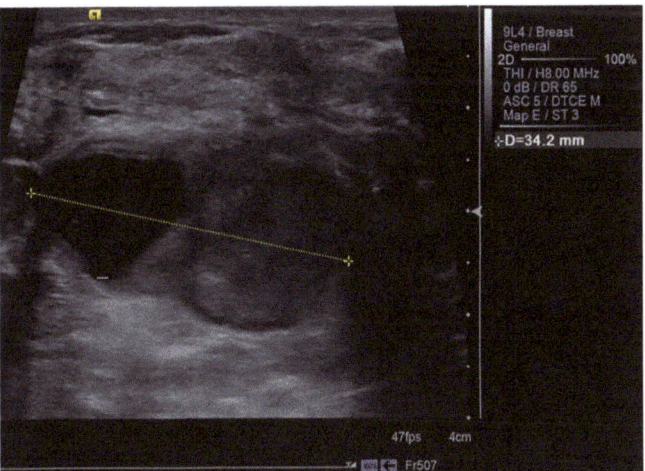

Fig. 9.34: B-mode ultrasound revealed a mixed mass with solid (slightly hypoechoic) and cystic component, well-defined outlines besides the median anterior part which is diffused with the adjacent tissue, wider than taller, absence of microcalcifications and posterior acoustic shadowing.

Color Doppler imaging has been shown in Figure 9.35.

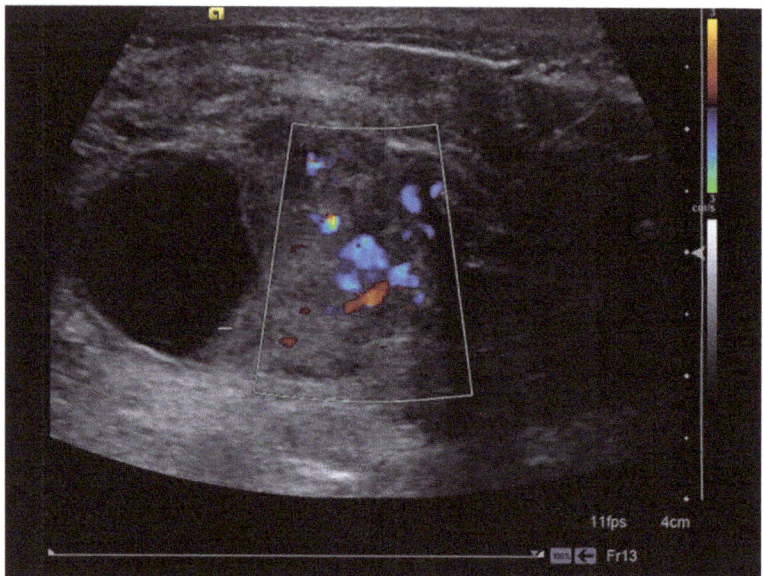

Fig. 9.35: Color Doppler revealed increased internal vascularity in the solid component.

Elasticity score has been shown in Figure 9.36.

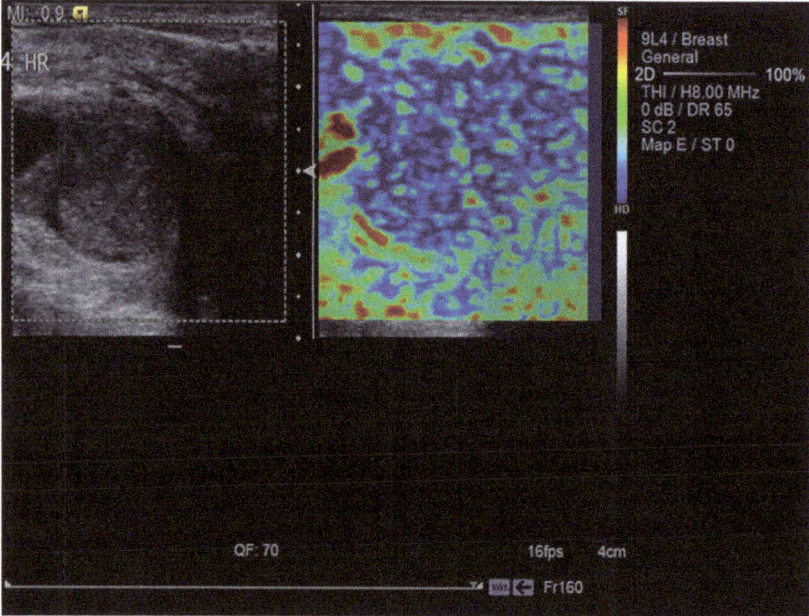

Fig. 9.36: Elasticity score = 2 (both soft and stiff areas) in the solid part of the lesion.

Calculation of strain ratio has been shown in Figure 9.37.

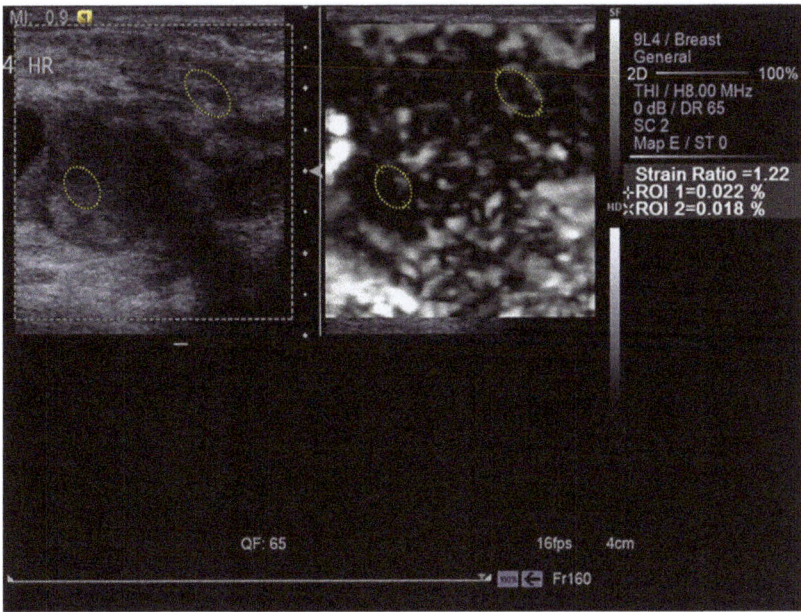

Fig. 9.37: Strain ratio was equal to 1.22 (ROI is placed inside the solid part of the lesion).

Grayscale VTI imaging has been shown in Figure 9.38.

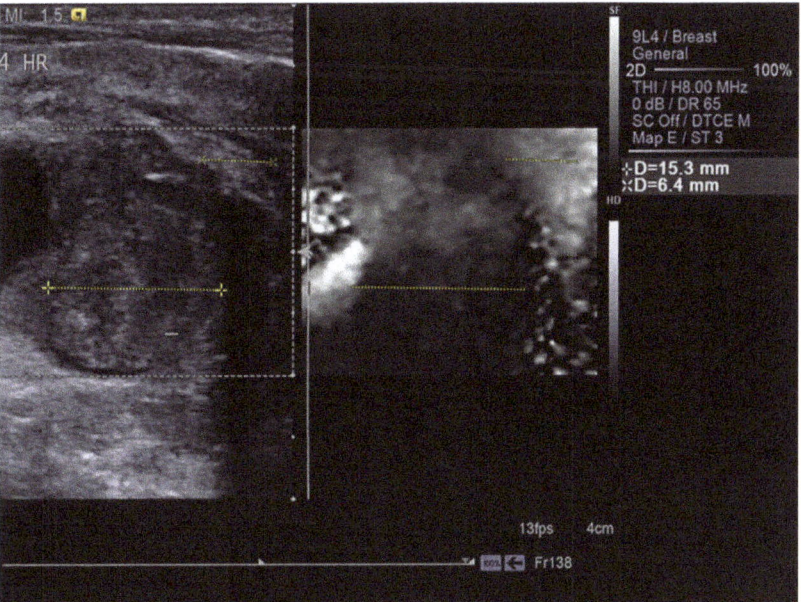

Fig. 9.38: "Equal stiffness" between the mass and the adjacent tissue.

VTQ value estimation inside the lesion has been shown in Figure 9.39.

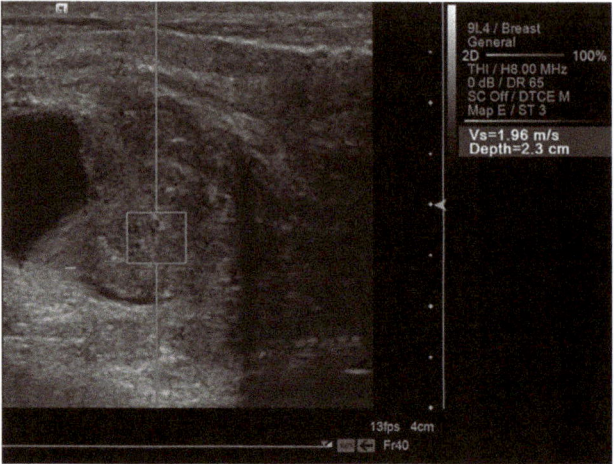

Fig. 9.39: VTQ value inside lesion solid part was 1.96 m/sec.

Pathology result has been shown in Figure 9.40.

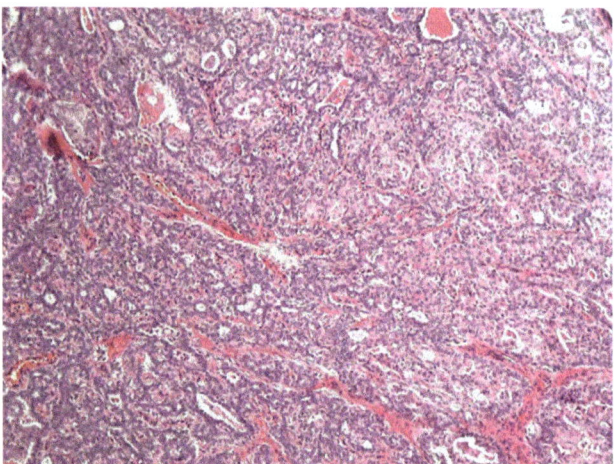

Fig. 9.40: Pathology result was adenomyoepithelioma. Myoepithelial cells layers surrounding epithelial lined spaces with tubular pattern A-EX100.

CONCLUSION

Elastographic findings were suggestive of benignity and in concordance with pathology result.

SUGGESTED READING

Gkali CA, Chalazonitis AN, Feida E, Dimitrakakis C, Sotiropoulou M. Breast Adenomyoepithelioma: Ultrasonography, Elastography, Digital Mammography, Contrast-Enhanced Digital Mammography, and Pathology Findings of This Rare Type of Breast Tumor. Ultrasound Q. 2015 Sep;31(3):185-8.

Chapter 9: Interpretation of Benign Breast Lesions | 85

CASE 7: A 42-year-old woman underwent B-mode ultrasound and elastography for evaluation of a known mass of the left breast at 5 o' clock.

Digital mammography findings have been shown in Figure 9.41.

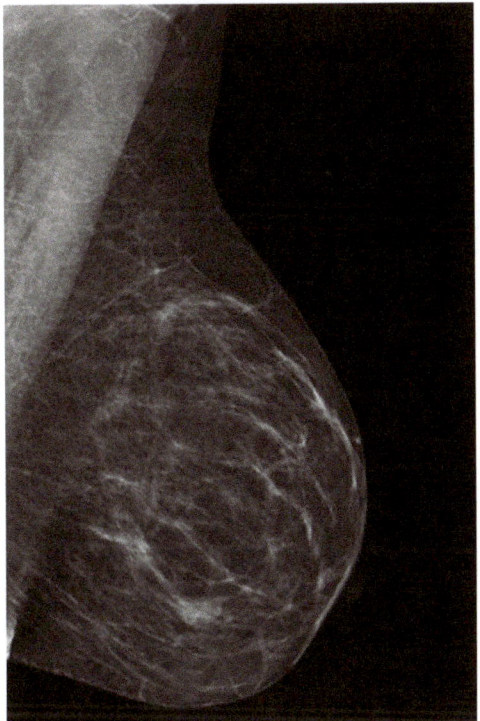

Fig. 9.41: MLO view of left breast depicts a partially circumscribed opacity.

B-mode ultrasound findings have been shown in Figure 9.42.

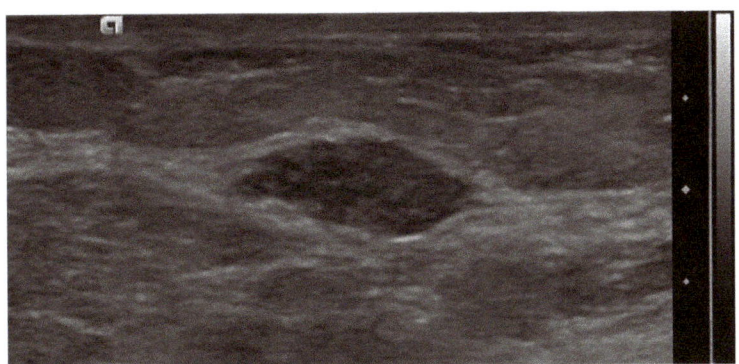

Fig. 9.42: B-mode ultrasound revealed an oval, hypoechoic, well-defined, encapsulated mass.

Color Doppler findings have been shown in Figure 9.43.

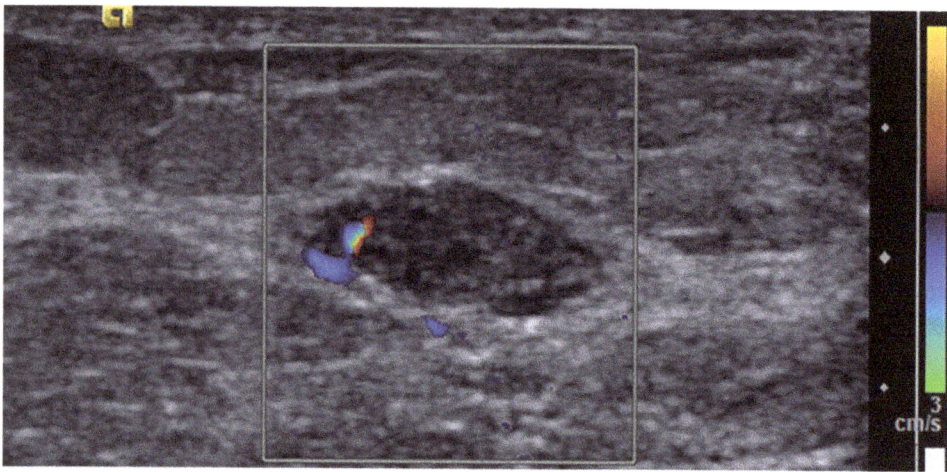

Fig. 9.43: Color Doppler revealed low, peripheral vascularity.

Calculation of strain ratio has been shown in Figure 9.44.

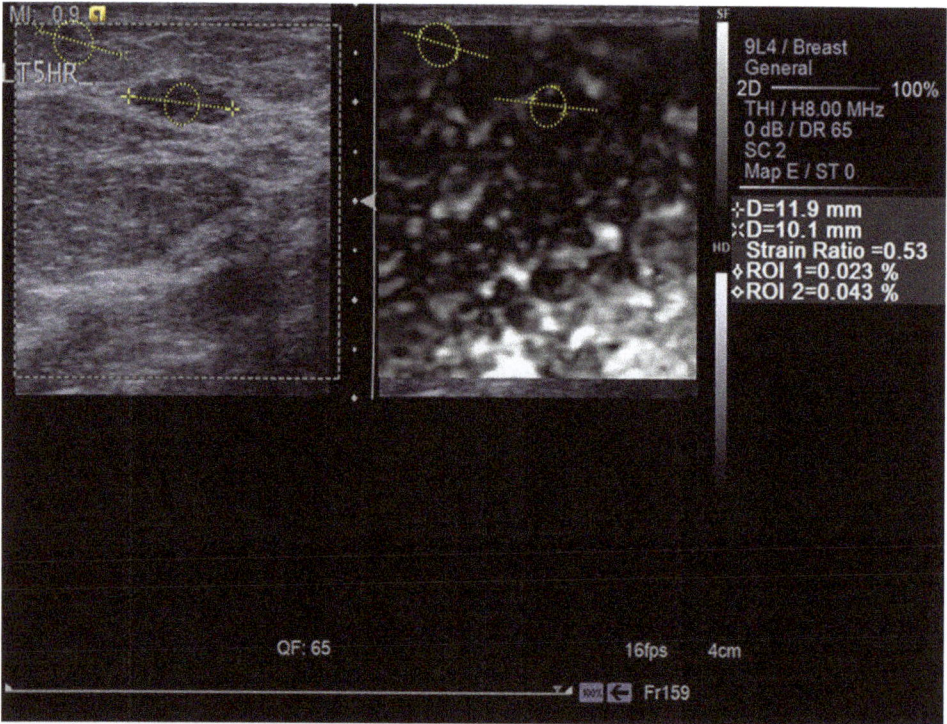

Fig. 9.44: Strain ratio was equal to 0.53.

Grayscale VTI imaging has been shown in Figure 9.45.

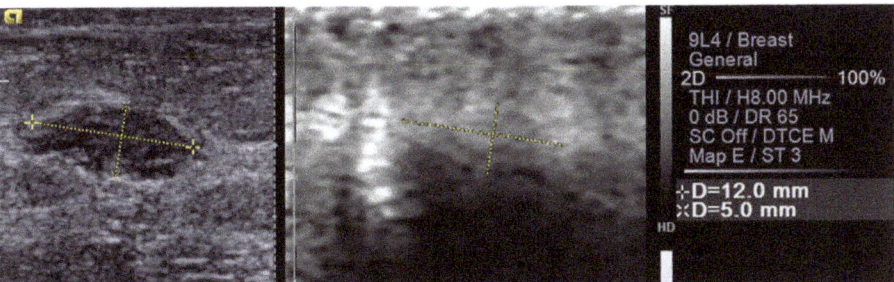

Fig. 9.45: VTI imaging depicted an equal stiffness mass to the surrounding breast tissue.

Color map VTI imaging has been shown in Figure 9.46.

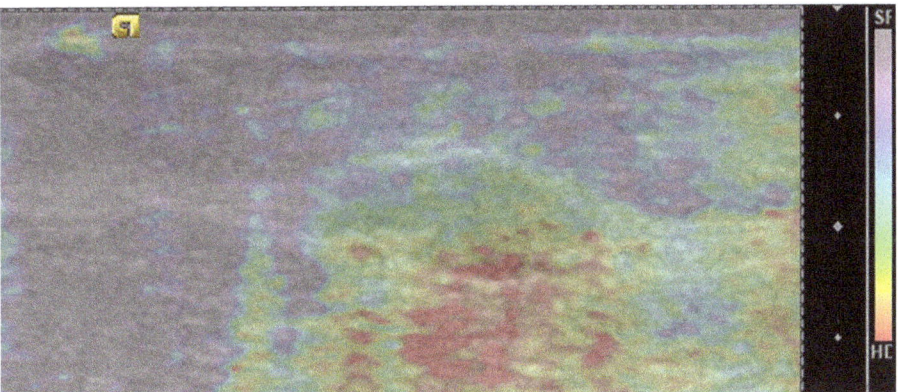

Fig. 9.46: The mass depicted mostly as green-purple.

VTQ value estimation inside the lesion has been shown in Figure 9.47.

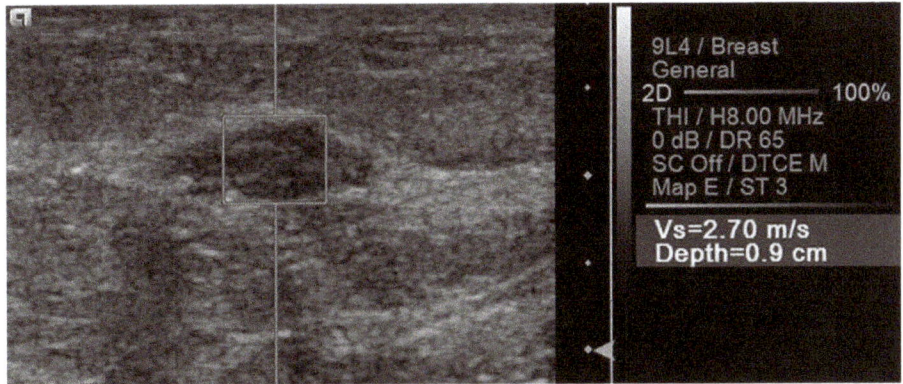

Fig. 9.47: VTQ value inside the lesion was equal to 2.70 m/sec.

VTQ value estimation in the adjacent tissue has been shown in Figure 9.48.

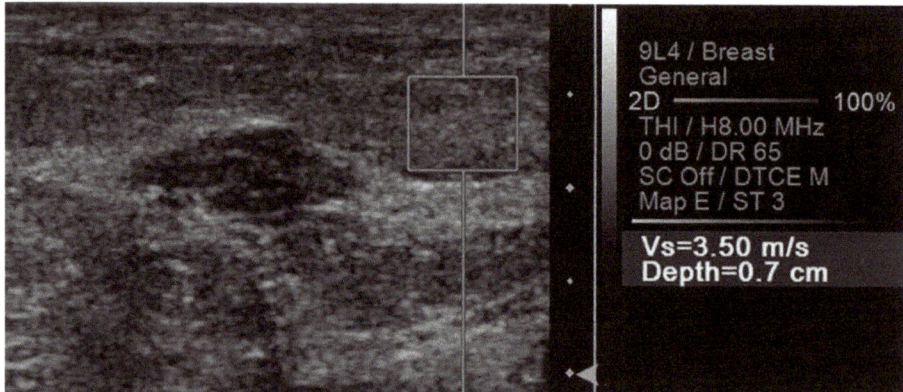

Fig. 9.48: VTQ value in the surrounding tissue (same depth) was equal to 3.50 m/sec.

Pathology result has been shown in Figure 9.49.

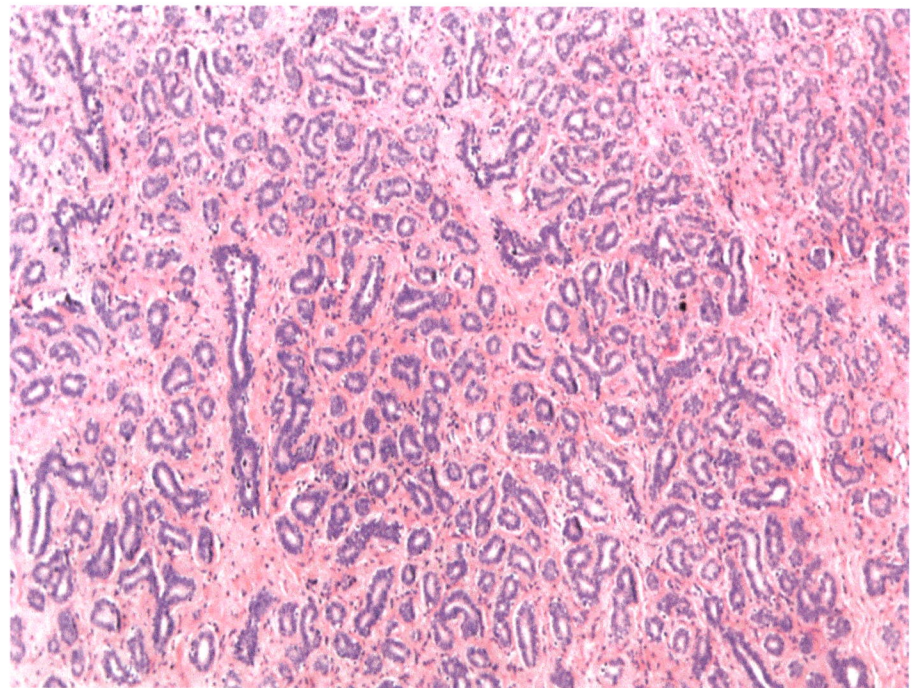

Fig. 9.49: Pathology result was tubular adenoma, a variant of fibroadenoma with florid adenosis.

CONCLUSION

Pathology and elastographic findings were in concordance.

Chapter 9: Interpretation of Benign Breast Lesions | 89

CASE 8: A 12-year-old girl was referred to our radiology department with a rapidly enlarging, painless mass of her right breast for 3 months duration.

Physical examination: Physical examination revealed a 15 cm × 13 cm, firm, not tender, mobile mass in the right breast.

B-mode ultrasound findings have been shown in Figure 9.50.

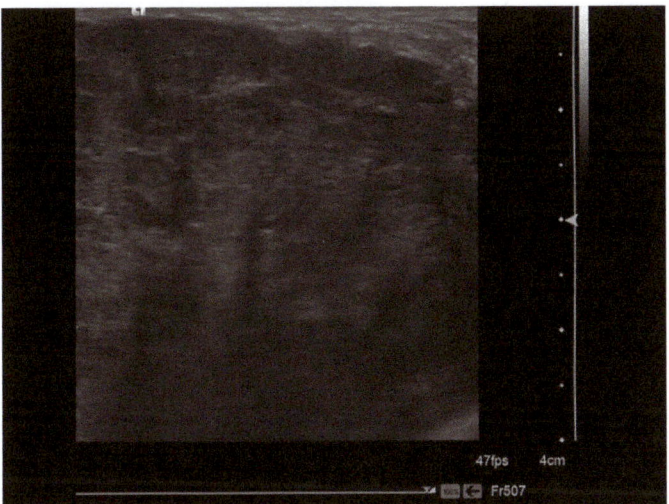

Fig. 9.50: B-mode US revealed an encapsulated, well-defined, slightly lobulated, iso- to hypoechoic mass with small cystic spaces. Neither microcalcifications nor posterior acoustic shadowing were present.

Color Doppler findings have been shown in Figure 9.51.

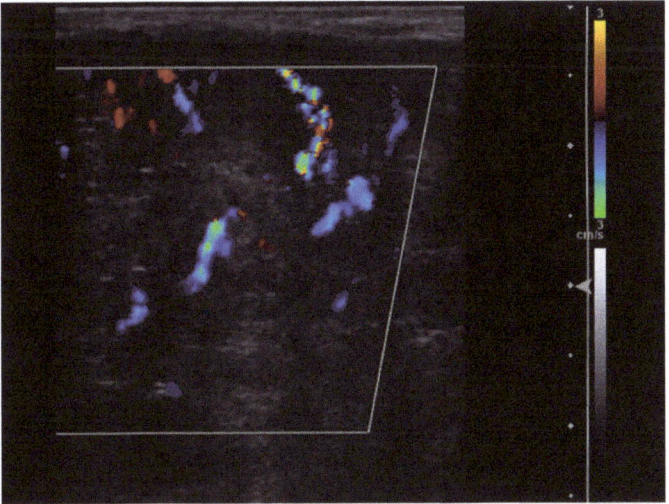

Fig. 9.51: Color Doppler revealed increased internal vascularity.

Grayscale VTI imaging has been shown in Figure 9.52.

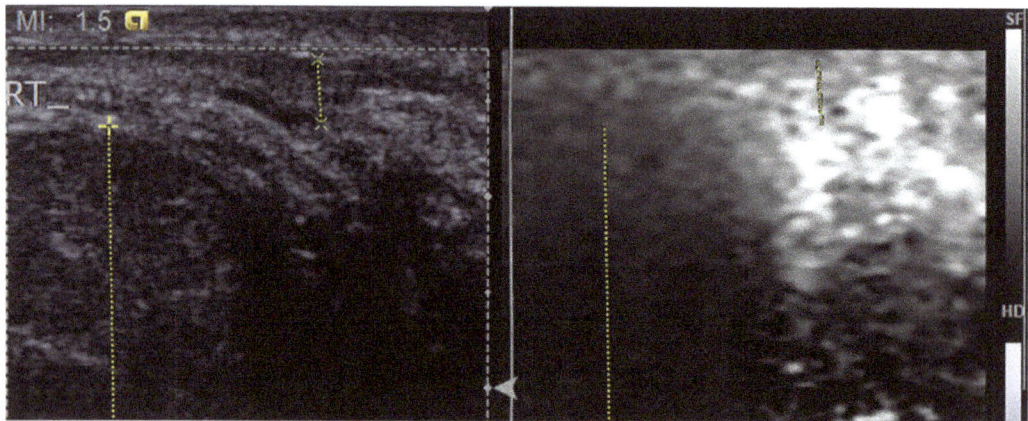

Fig. 9.52: VTI image revealed a mass with equal stiffness with the adjacent tissue.

Color map VTI imaging has been shown in Figure 9.53.

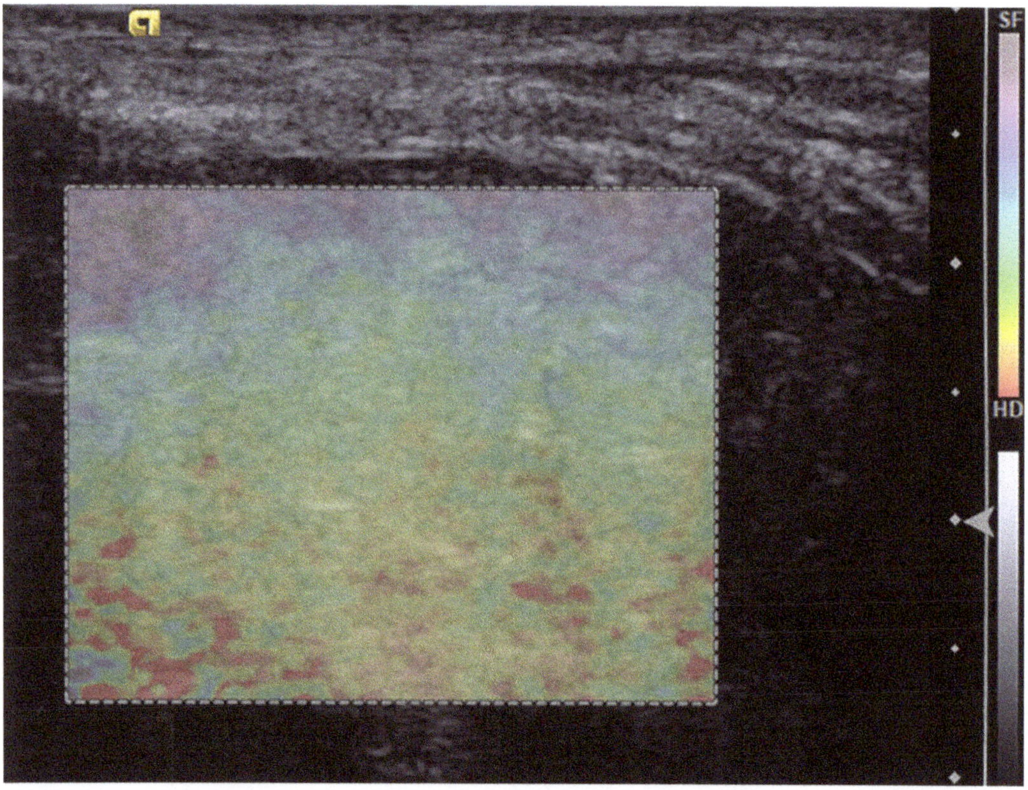

Fig. 9.53: The mass depicted as mostly green (soft) with yellow-red areas (stiff).

VTQ value inside the lesion has been shown in Figures 9.54A and B.

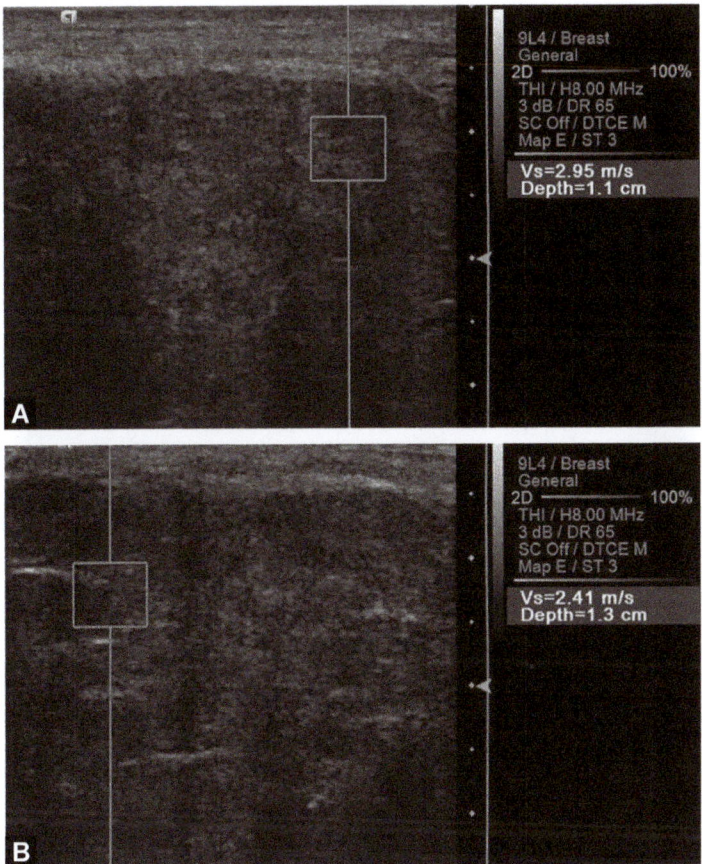

Figs. 9.54A and B: VTQ values were calculated inside the lesion with maximum Vs = 2.95 m/sec.

VTQ value in the surrounding tissue has been shown in Figure 9.55.

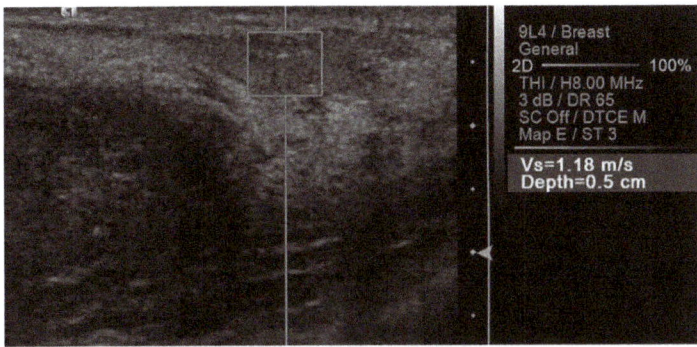

Fig. 9.55: VTQ value within the adjacent normal tissue was 1.18 m/sec.

The patient was subjected to fine-needle aspiration cytology (FNAC) of the breast lump with pathology suggesting fibroadenoma.

Following diagnostic evaluation and FNAC, surgical excisional biopsy was performed (Figs. 9.56A and B).

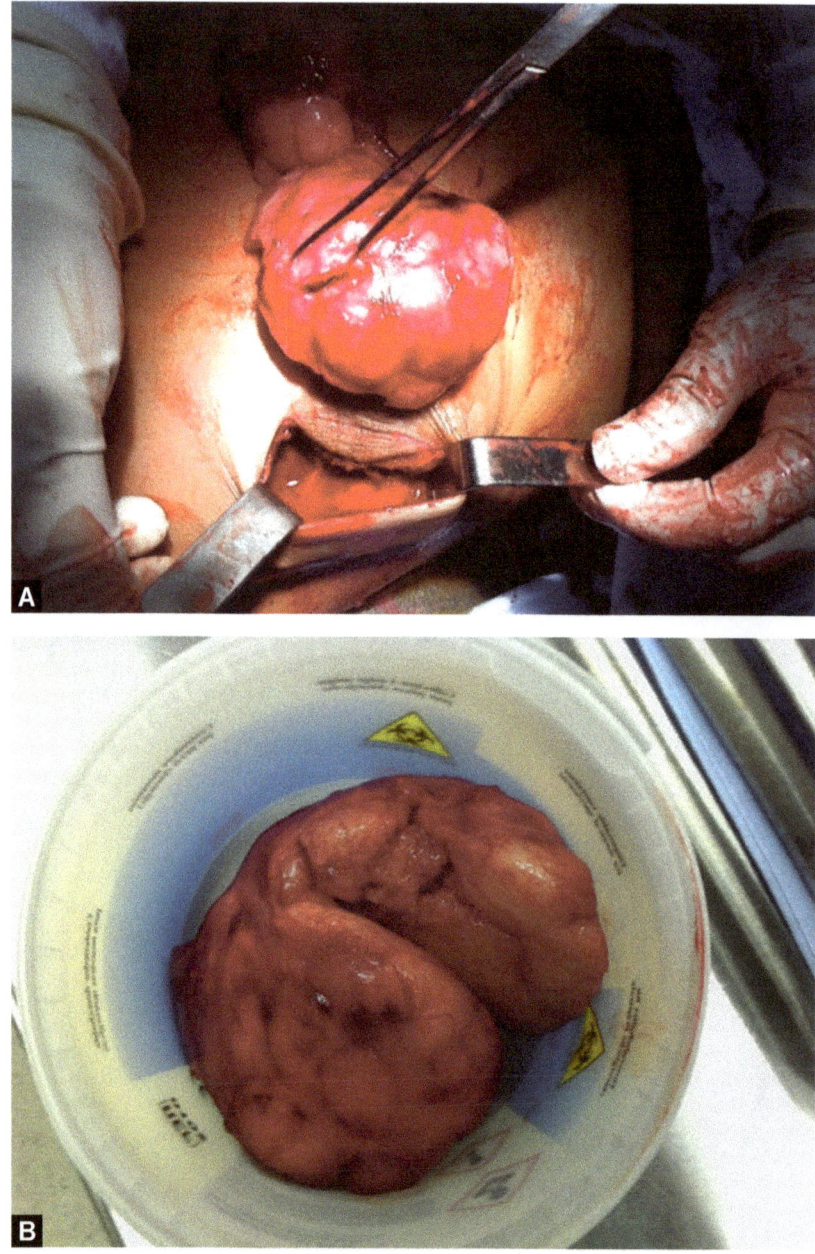

Figs. 9.56A and B: Intraoperative image of the mass.

Pathology result has been shown in Figure 9.57.

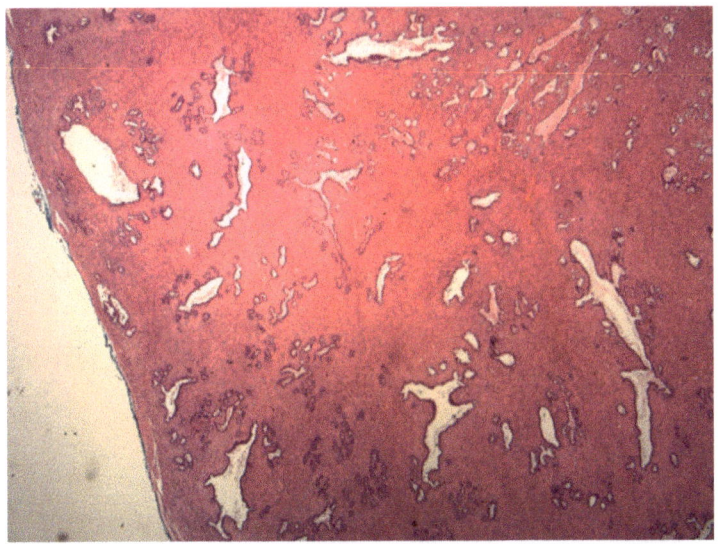

Fig. 9.57: Pathology result was juvenile fibroadenoma with pericanalicular architecture, mild epithelial hyperplasia and stromal cellularity (hematoxylin-eosin).

Postoperative image has been shown in Figure 9.58.

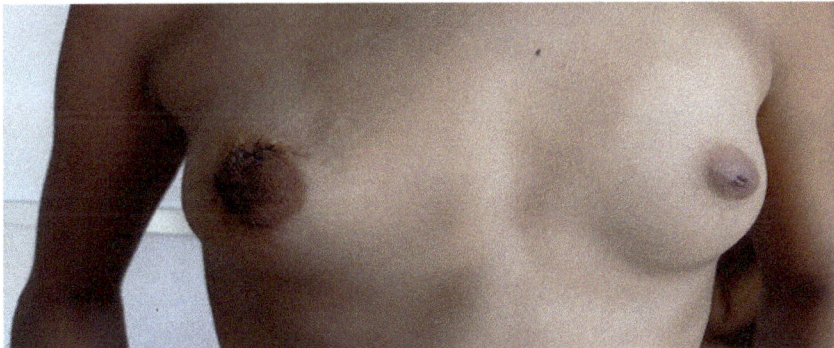

Fig. 9.58: Postoperative image of breasts.

CONCLUSION

According to the combined results of strain and acoustic radiation force impulse (ARFI) elastography, the mass was evaluated as probably benign.

In this case, there were some difficulties. One of them was that the lesion was large enough and the surrounding tissue was displaced. This made difficult to place the ROI in the adjacent tissue, so the strain ratio could be calculated. It was also difficult to compare the ROIs in VTI grayscale imaging.

Section 6: Interpretation of Benign and Malignant Breast Lesions

CASE 9: A 45-year-old referred for a palpable mass of the left breast.

Physical examination: Physical examination revealed a painless, palpable mass in the outer part of left breast.

Digital mammography findings have been shown in Figure 9.59.

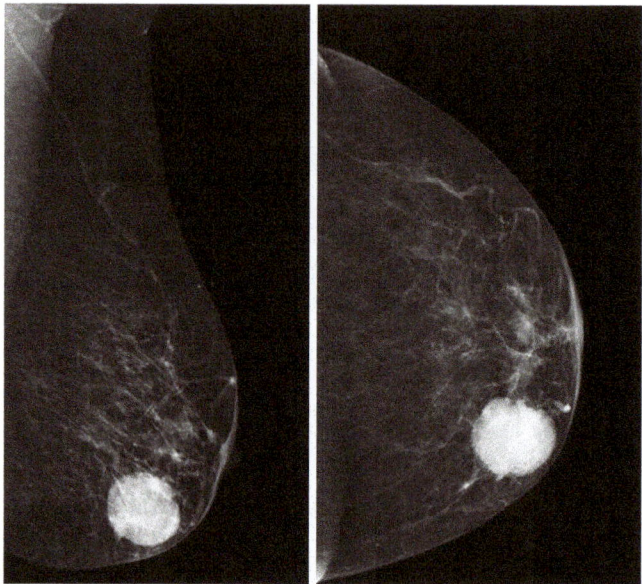

Fig. 9.59: MLO and CC views of left breast revealed an enlarged, partially circumscribed mass.

B-mode ultrasound findings have been shown in Figure 9.60.

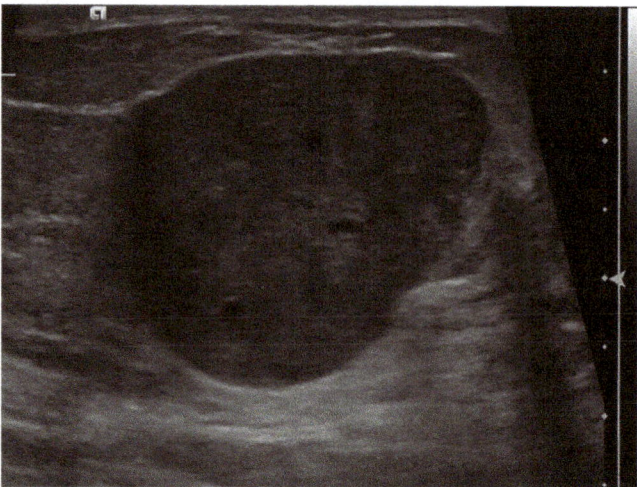

Fig. 9.60: B-mode revealed a slightly hypoechoic, well-circumscribed, with cystic spaces mass.

Color Doppler findings have been shown in Figure 9.61.

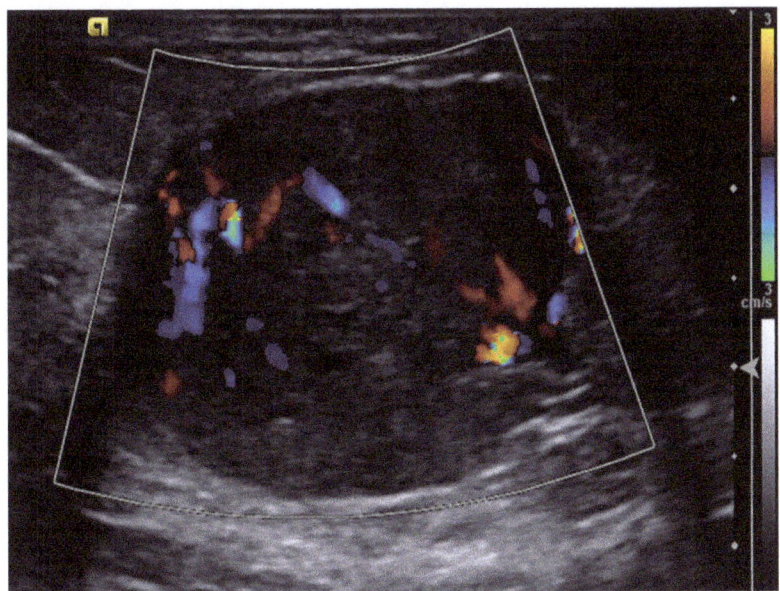

Fig. 9.61: Increased internal vascularity.

Strain ratio calculation has been shown in Figure 9.62.

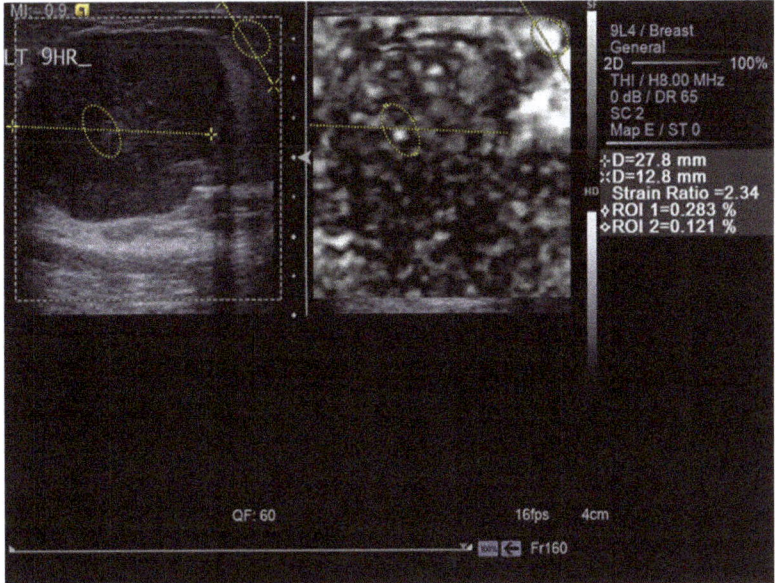

Fig. 9.62: Strain ratio (SR) = 2.34.

Elasticity score has been shown in Figure 9.63.

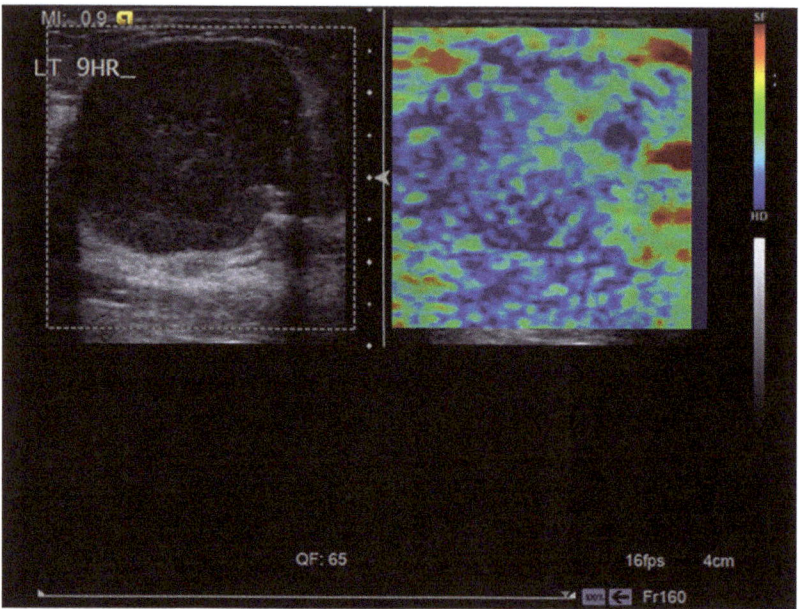

Fig. 9.63: Elasticity score = 2.

Color map VTI imaging has been shown in Figure 9.64.

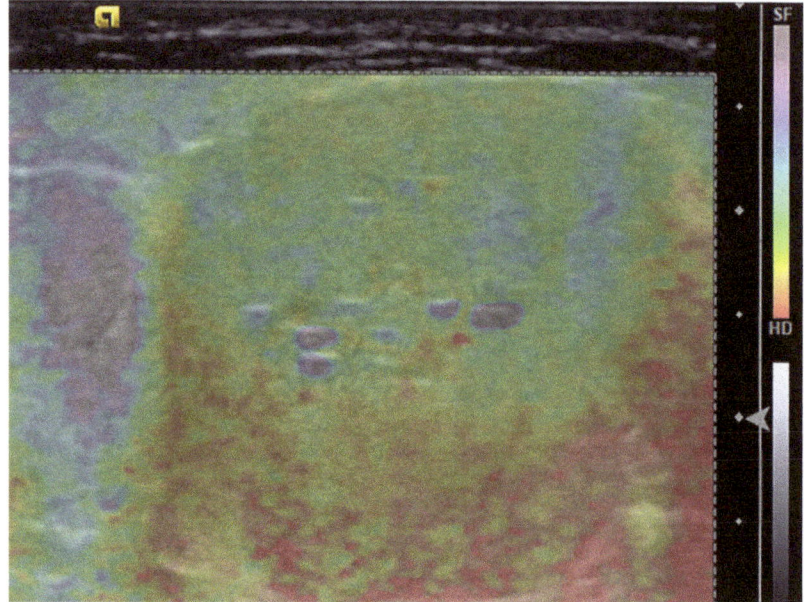

Fig. 9.64: The lesion appears mostly purple-blue-green (soft).

VTQ value estimation inside the lesion has been shown in Figure 9.65.

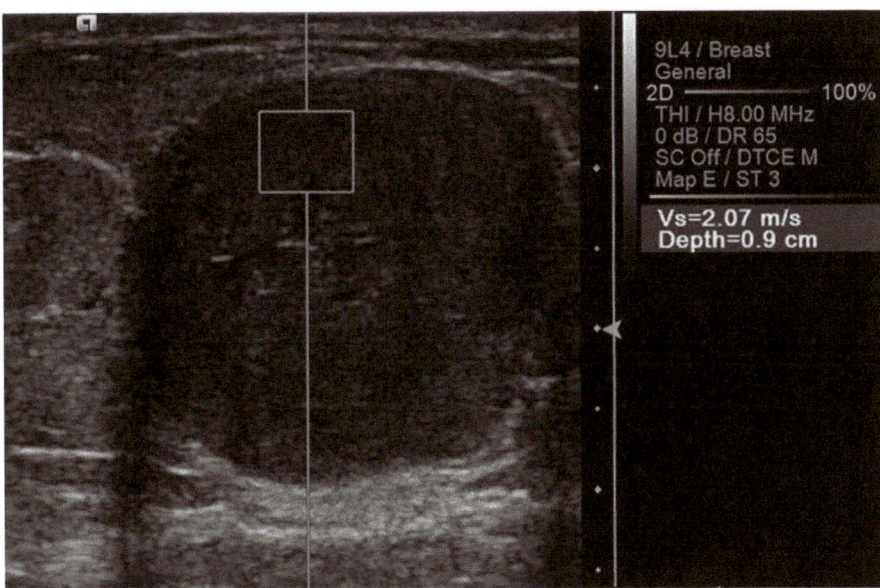

Fig. 9.65: Vs = 2.07 m/sec.

VTQ value estimation in the adjacent tissue has been shown in Figure 9.66.

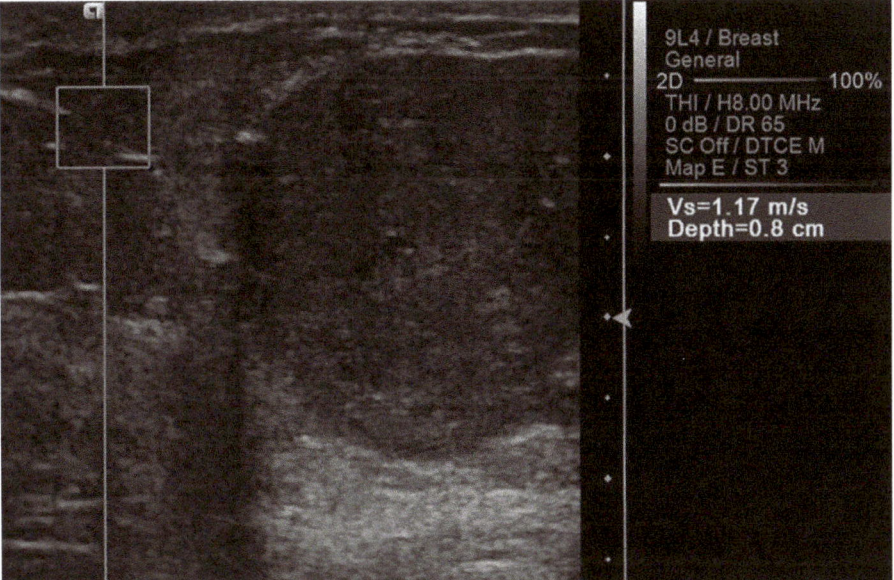

Fig. 9.66: Vs = 1.17 m/sec (same depth).

Pathology result has been shown in Figure 9.67.

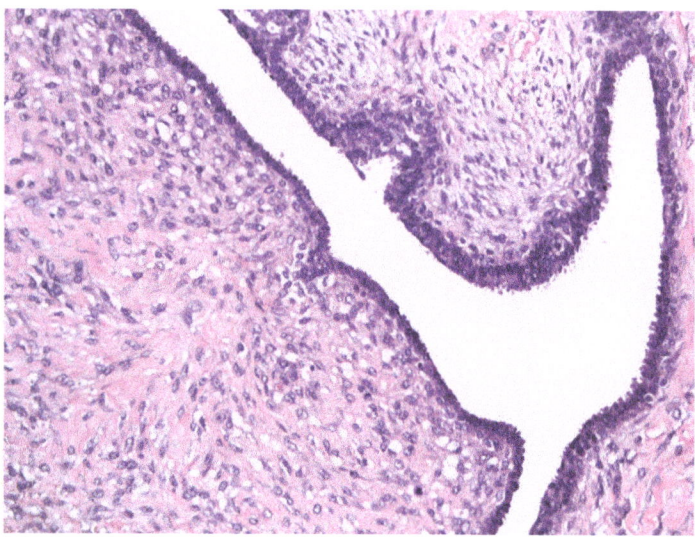

Fig. 9.67: Pathology result was phyllodes tumor (long clefts with hypercellular mesenchymal component).

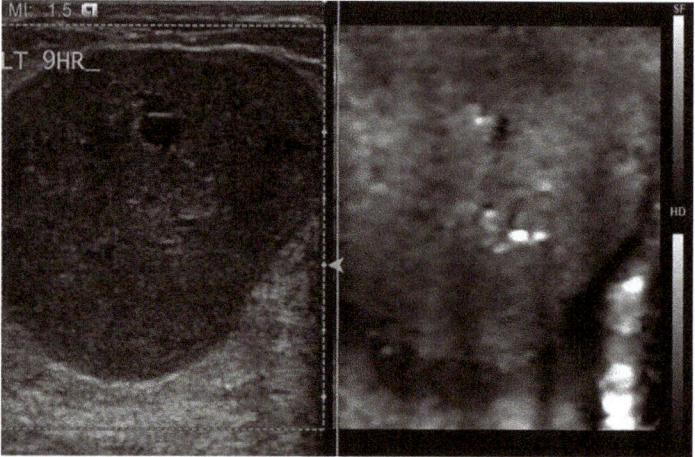

Fig. 9.68: Notice: In this VTI image you can observe that the cystic space of the mass appears the typical bull's eye artifact.

CONCLUSION

Elastographic findings were suggestive of benignity and in concordance with pathology result.

In this case, it is important to mention that the grayscale VTI image was difficult to be evaluated as the mass was large enough and the comparison of two ROIs between the mass and surrounding tissue was impossible (Fig. 9.68).

CHAPTER 10: Interpretation of Malignant Breast Lesions

Christina An. Gkali

CASE 1: A 45-year-old woman was referred to our radiology department with a palpable lesion of the right breast for 2 months.

Physical examination revealed a single mass in the lower outer quadrant of the right breast. No lymph node enlargement was detected.

Digital mammography findings have been shown in Figures 10.1 and 10.2.

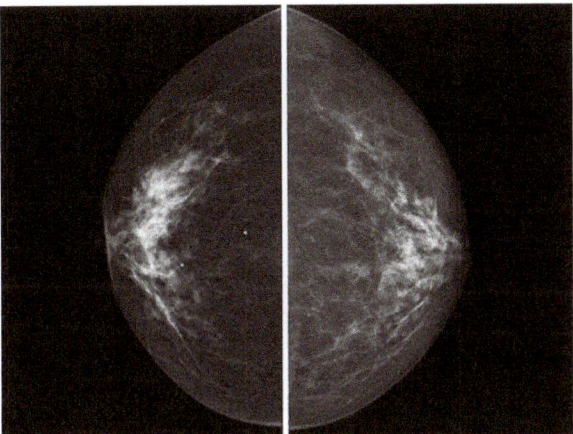

Fig. 10.1: Craniocaudal (CC) digital mammography images evaluated as breast imaging-reporting and data system (BI-RADS) IV classification on the right breast.

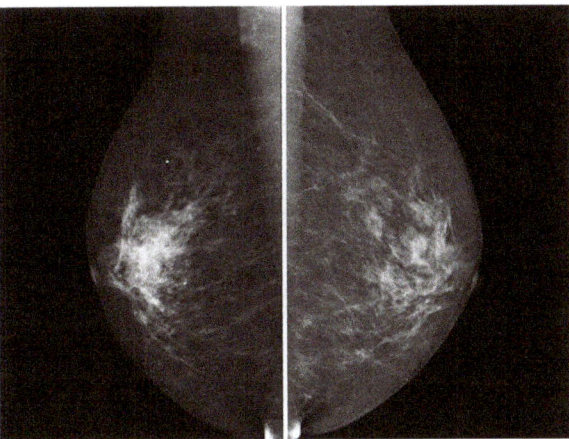

Fig. 10.2: Mediolateral oblique (MLO) view evaluated as BI-RADS IV classification on the right breast.

B-mode ultrasound findings have been shown in Figure 10.3.

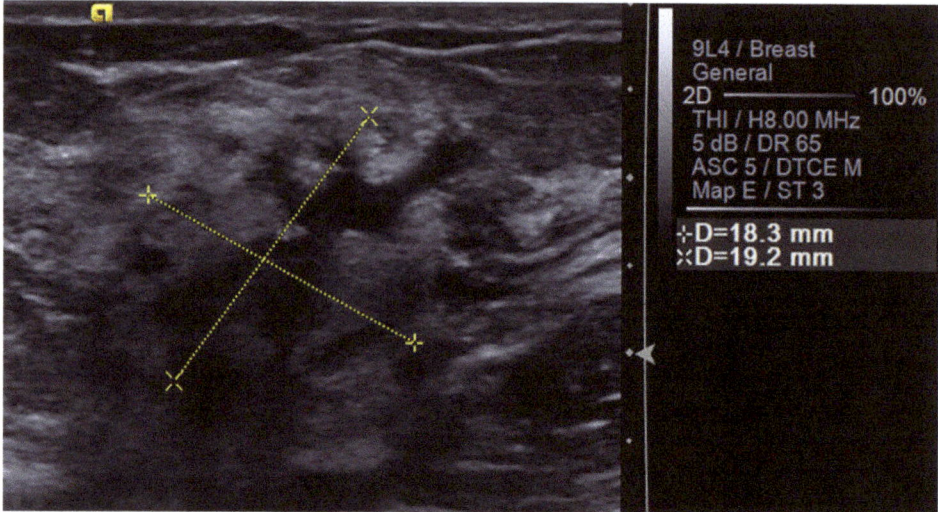

Fig. 10.3: B-mode ultrasound (US) revealed a solitary, hypoechoic mass with echogenic boundary, irregular in shape with indistinct margins. Neither microcalcifications nor posterior acoustic shadowing were present.

Color Doppler findings have been shown in Figure 10.4.

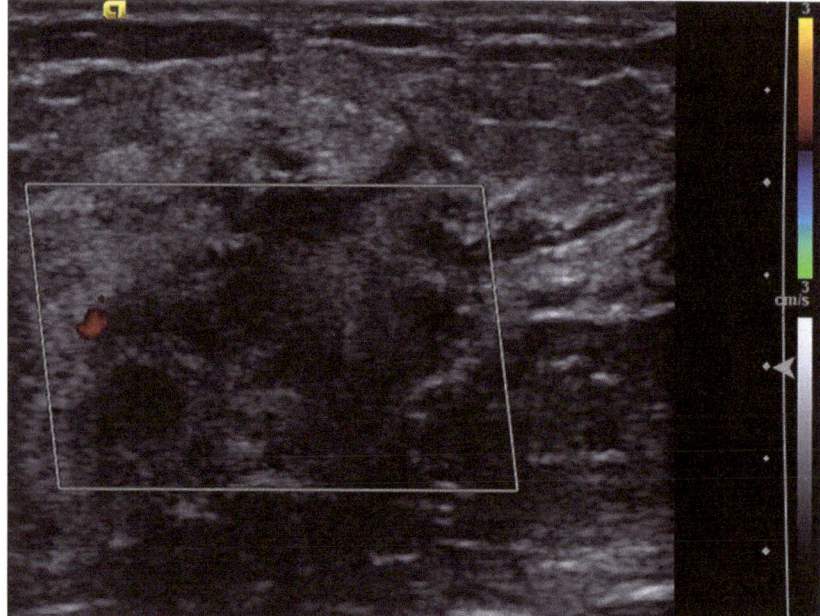

Fig. 10.4: Color Doppler revealed no increased internal vascularity.

Strain imaging—calculation of strain ratio has been shown in Figure 10.5.

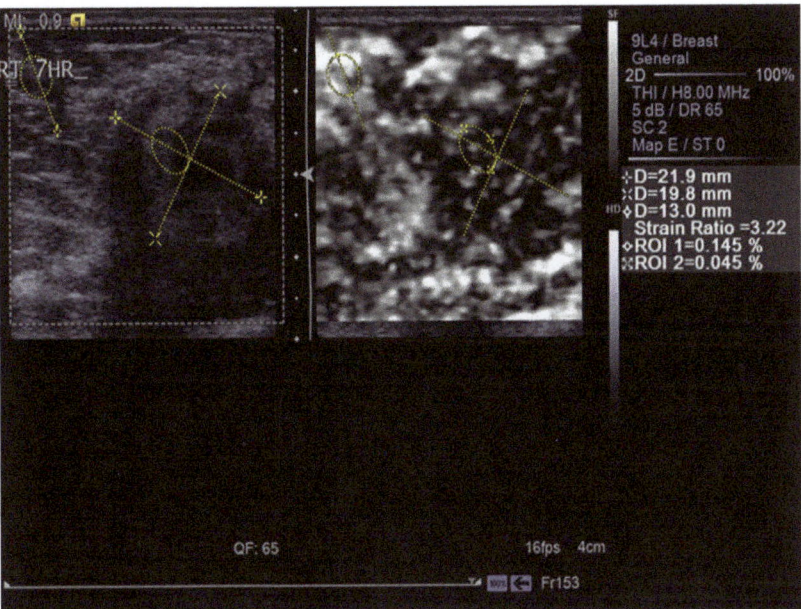

Fig. 10.5: Strain ratio was calculated and equal to 3.22.

Elasticity score has been shown in Figure 10.6.

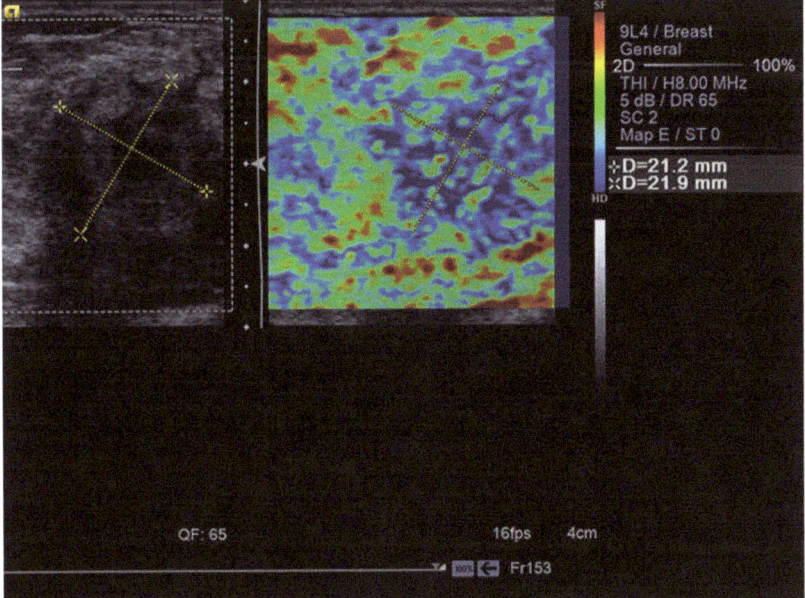

Fig. 10.6: Elasticity score was 3.

Virtual touch quantification (VTQ) value inside the lesion has been shown in Figure 10.7.

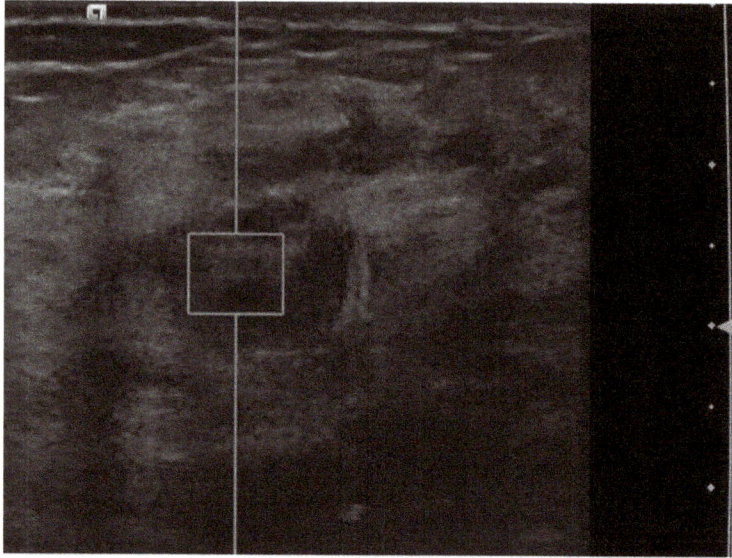

Fig. 10.7: VTQ value inside the lesion was 6.98 m/sec.

Pathology result has been shown in Figures 10.8 and 10.9.

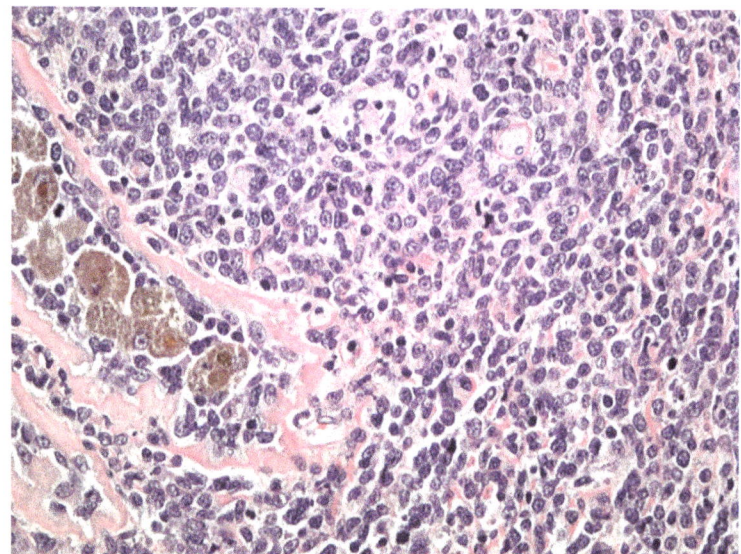

Fig. 10.8: Pathology result was primary non-Hodgkin's lymphoma B-cell origin of the breast. Lymphoma cells infiltrate in diffuse pattern fibrofatty breast tissue (A-E × 200).

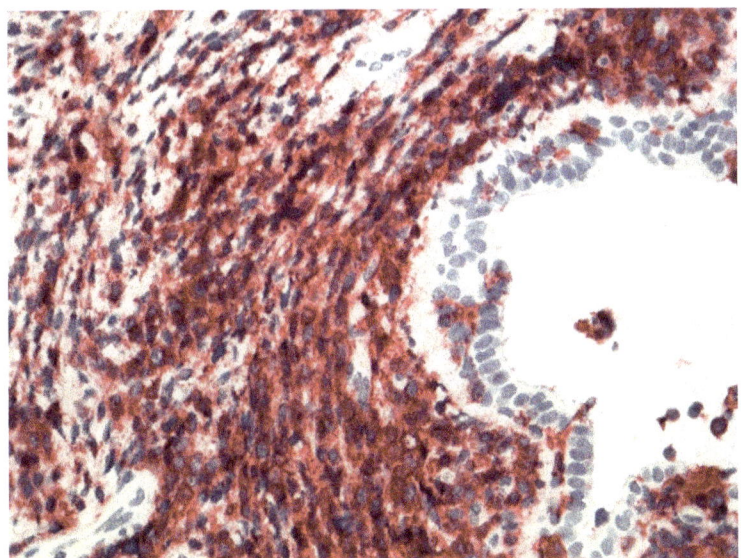

Fig. 10.9: Tumor cells were strongly immunoreactive for L26 showing B-cell origin. Periductal infiltration (CD20 × 400).

CONCLUSION

Elastographic findings were indicative of malignancy and in concordance with pathology findings.

0.15% of malignant breast neoplasms are lymphomas. Breast, primarily, is involved in less than 0.5% of all malignant lymphomas. The diagnosis of primary breast lymphoma is limited to patients with no evidence of systemic lymphoma or leukemia when the breast lesion is detected.

CASE 2: A 71-year-old woman referred for screening mammography.

Digital mammography findings have been shown in Figure 10.10.

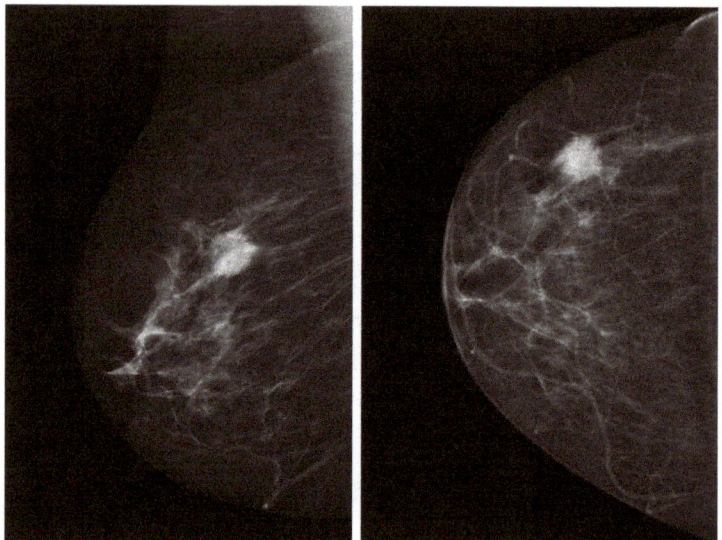

Fig. 10.10: MLO and CC views of right breast depict a spiculated, irregular high-density mass in the upper outer quadrant.

B-mode ultrasound findings have been shown in Figures 10.11 and 10.12.

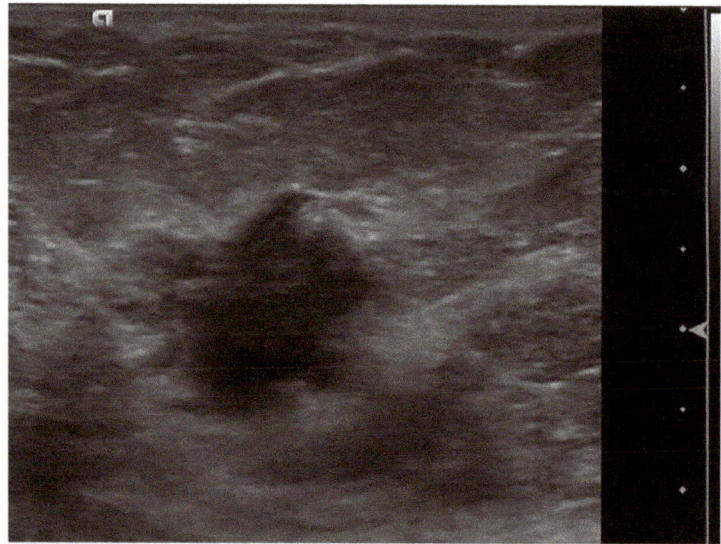

Fig. 10.11: B-mode ultrasound revealed a marked hypoechoic mass, with indistinct margins and spiculations.

Chapter 10: Interpretation of Malignant Breast Lesions

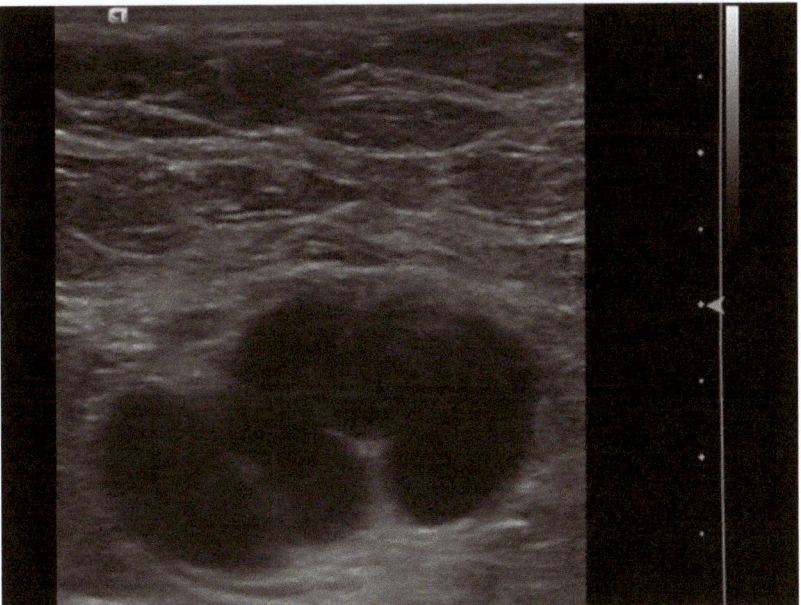

Fig. 10.12: Notice also the present of axillary lymph node with markedly thickened lymph node cortex and loss of the normal fatty hilum.

Grayscale strain imaging has been shown in Figure 10.13.

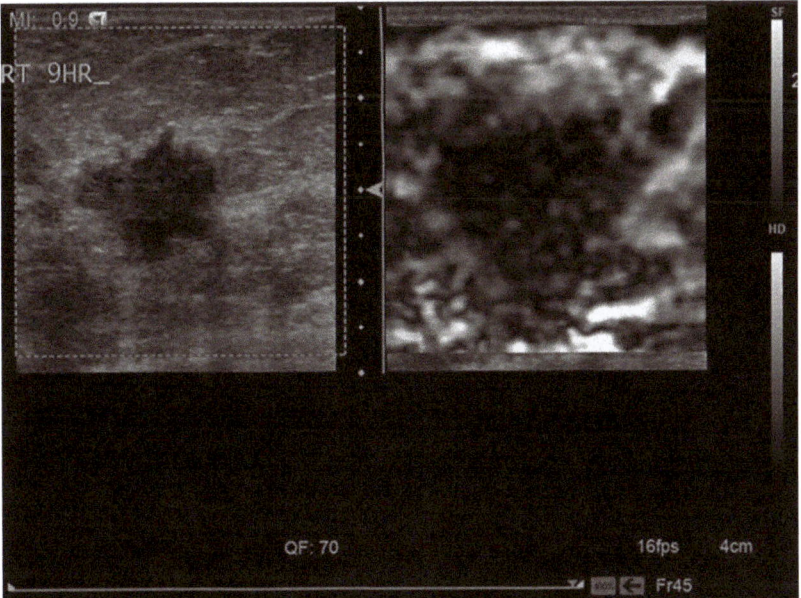

Fig. 10.13: The lesion appears darker (= stiffer) than the surrounding tissue and bigger than in B-mode image (E/B >1).

Strain ratio calculation has been shown in Figure 10.14.

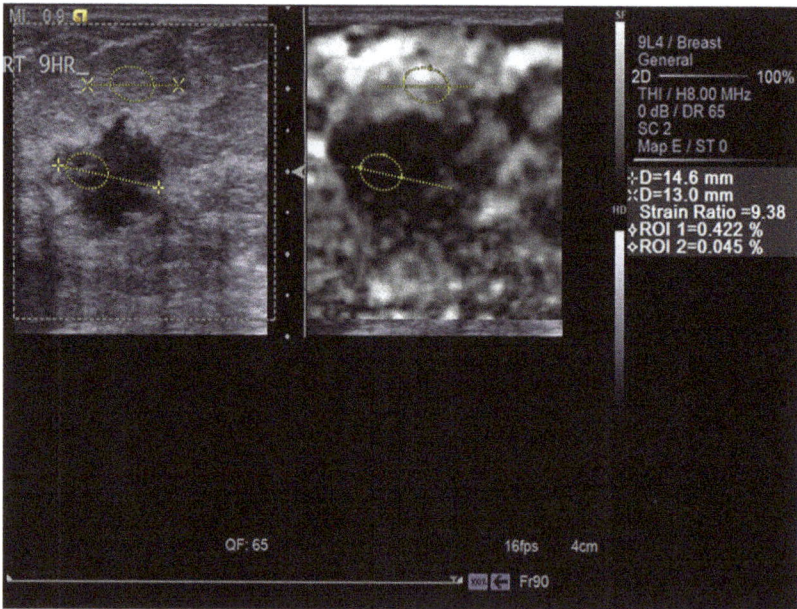

Fig. 10.14: Strain ratio was 9.38 (very high).

Elasticity score has been shown in Figure 10.15.

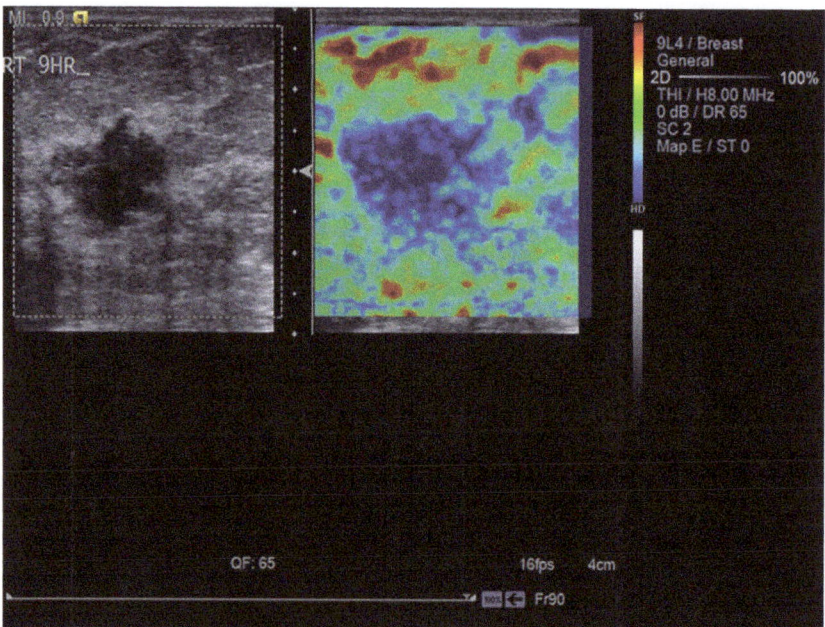

Fig. 10.15: Elasticity score is 4 (the entire lesion is stiff).

Virtual touch imaging (VTI)-grayscale imaging has been shown in Figure 10.16.

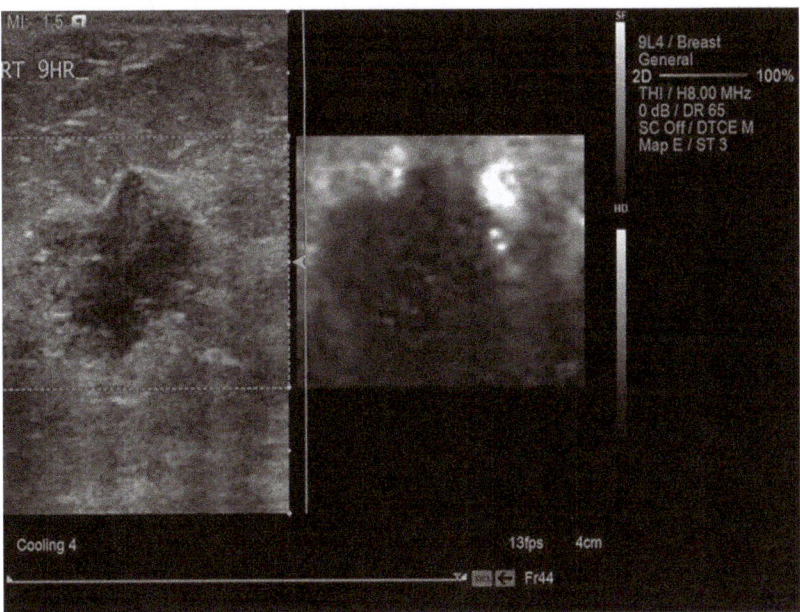

Fig. 10.16: The lesion appears stiffer than the surrounding tissue.

Color map VTI imaging has been shown in Figure 10.17.

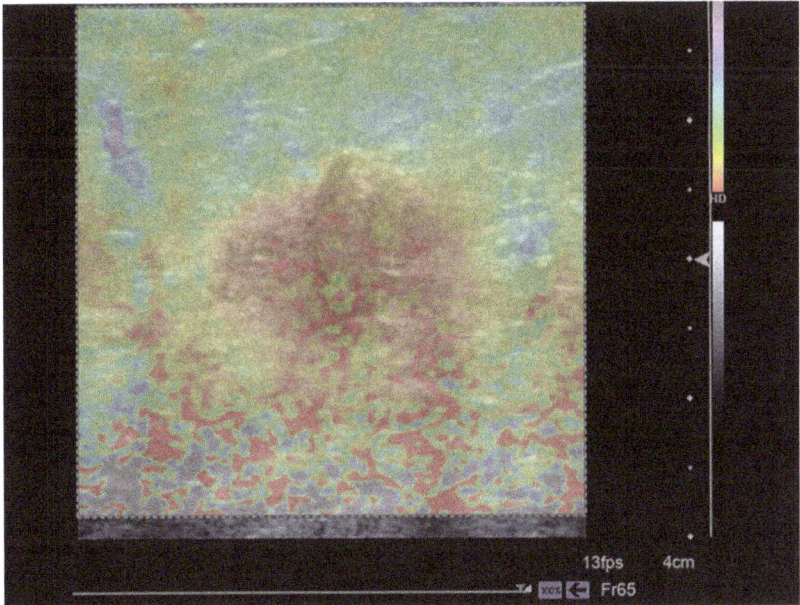

Fig. 10.17: The mass is red (= stiff).

VTQ value estimation has been shown in Figure 10.18.

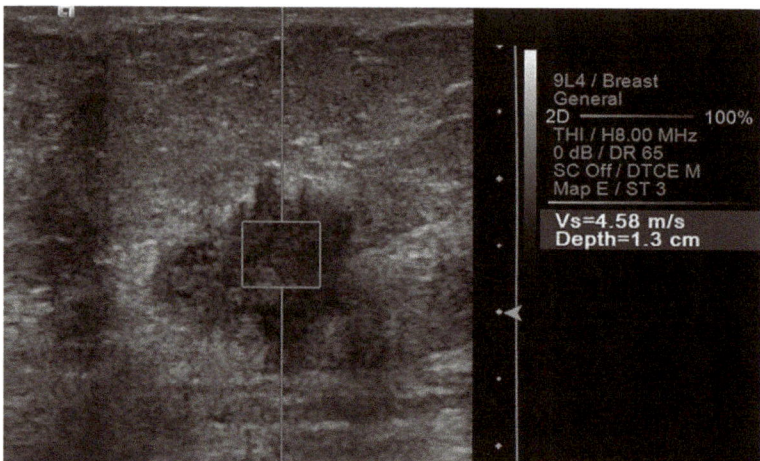

Fig. 10.18: Vs = 4.58 m/sec.

Pathology result has been shown in Figure 10.19.

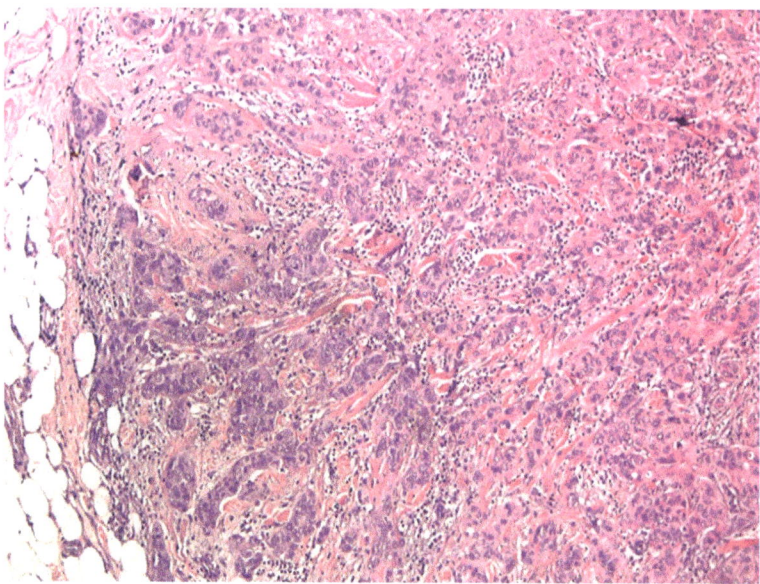

Fig. 10.19: Pathology result was coexistent invasive and intraepithelial ductal carcinoma, with ten infiltrated lymph nodes.

CONCLUSION

Elastographic findings were indicative of malignancy and in concordance with pathology result.

CASE 3: A 68-year-old woman.

B-mode ultrasound findings have been shown in Figure 10.20.

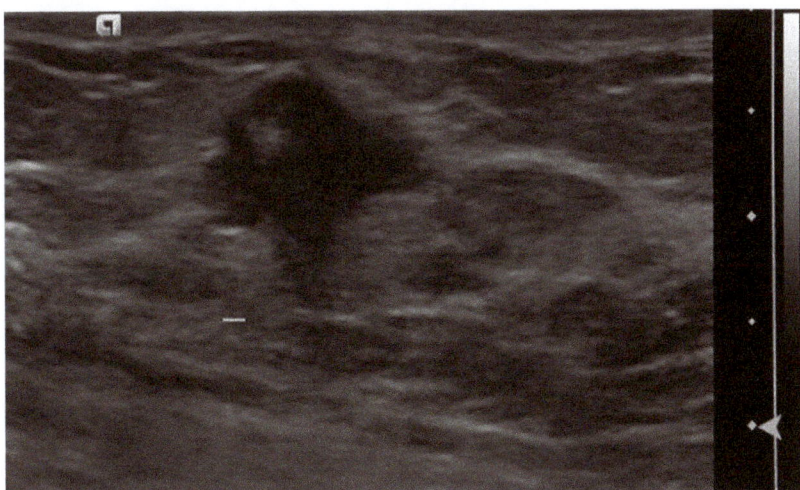

Fig. 10.20: B-mode ultrasound revealed a marked hypoechoic mass with indistinct margins and spiculations.

Strain ratio calculation has been shown in Figure 10.21.

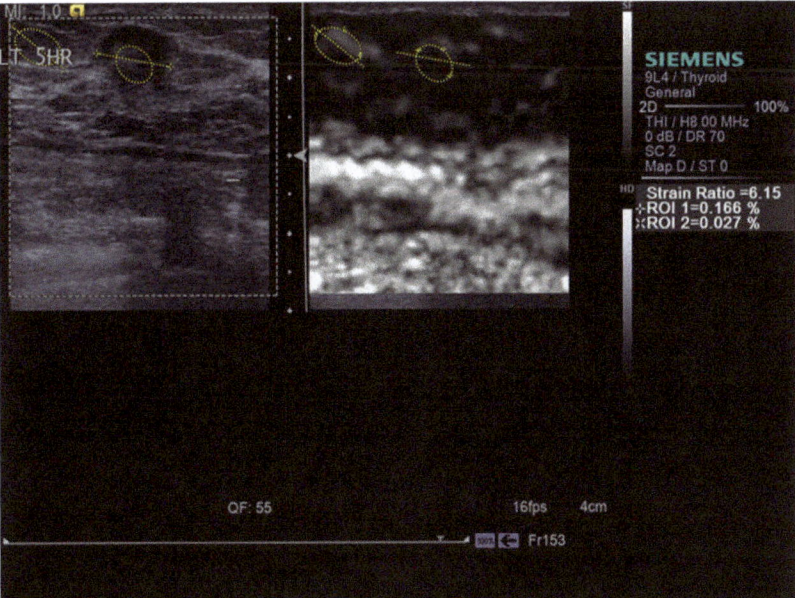

Fig. 10.21: Strain ratio was equal to 6.15.

Elasticity score has been shown in Figure 10.22.

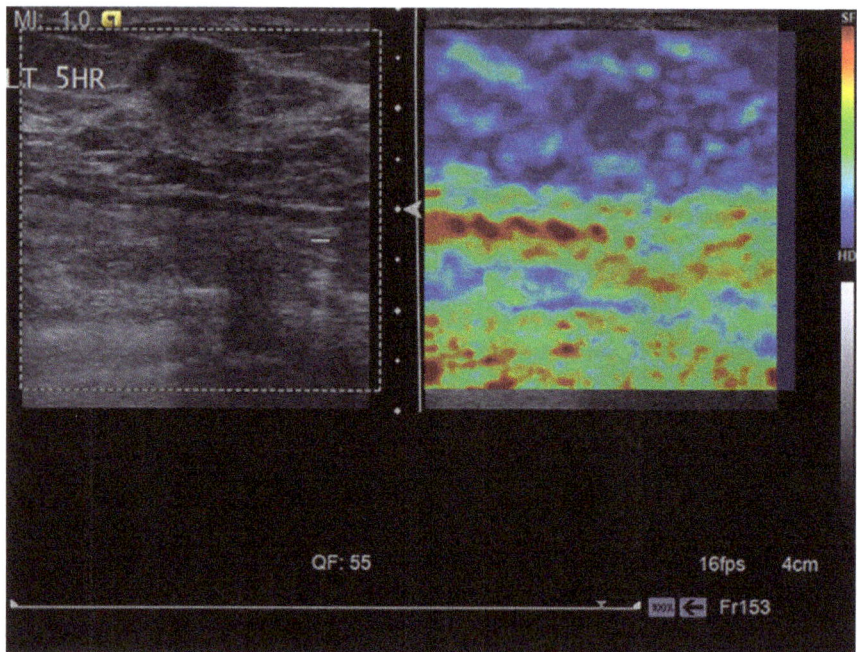

Fig. 10.22: Elasticity score = 5 (the entire lesion and surrounding tissue are stiff).

Grayscale VTI imaging has been shown in Figure 10.23.

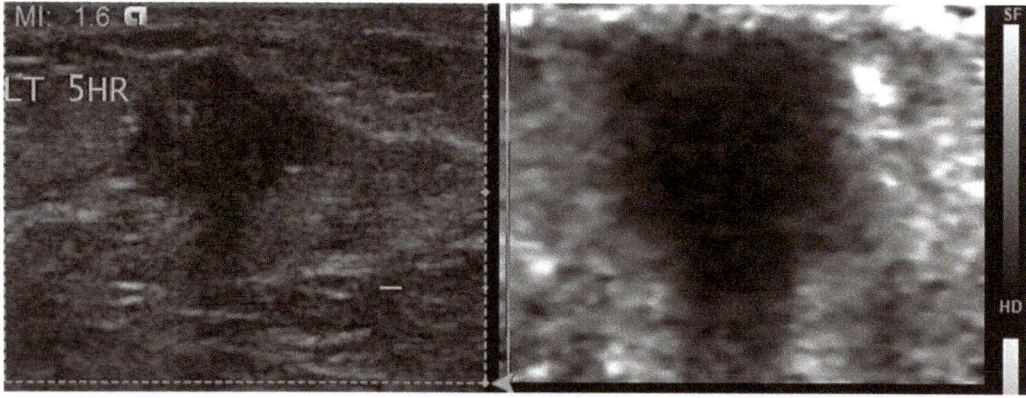

Fig. 10.23: The lesion appears stiffer than the surrounding tissue.

Color map VTI imaging has been shown in Figure 10.24.

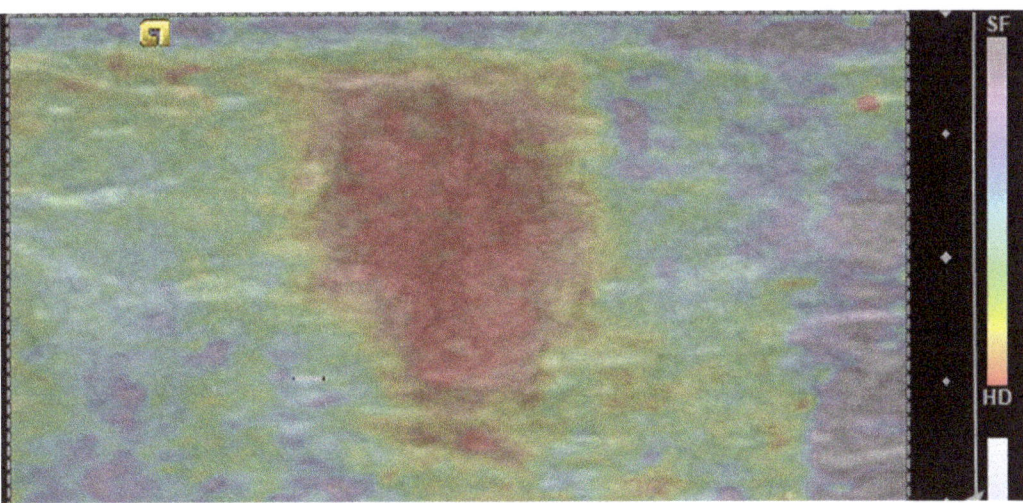

Fig. 10.24: The lesion is totally red (= stiff).

VTQ value estimation inside the lesion has been shown in Figure 10.25.

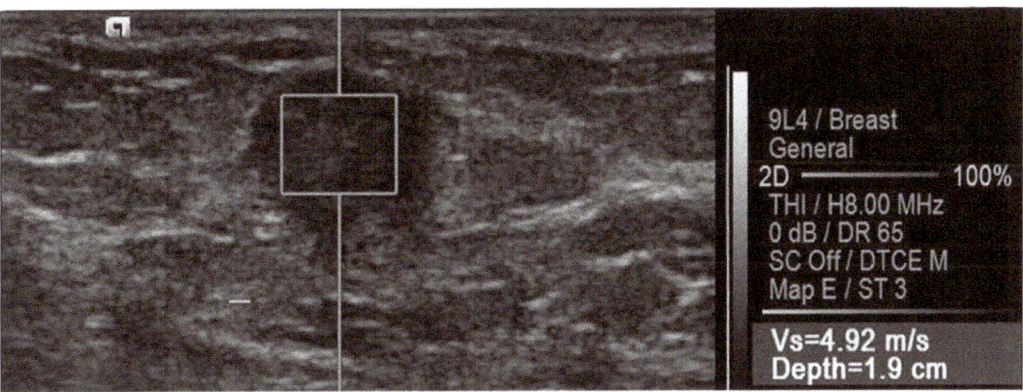

Fig. 10.25: Vs inside the lesion is estimated 4.92 m/sec.

VTQ value in the surrounding tissue has been shown in Figure 10.26.

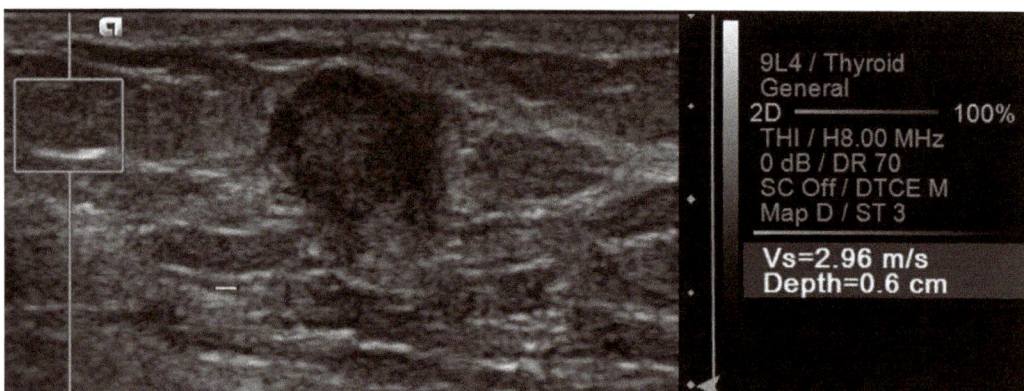

Fig. 10.26: Vs inside the surrounding tissue (same depth) is equal to 2.96 m/sec.

Pathology result has been shown in Figure 10.27.

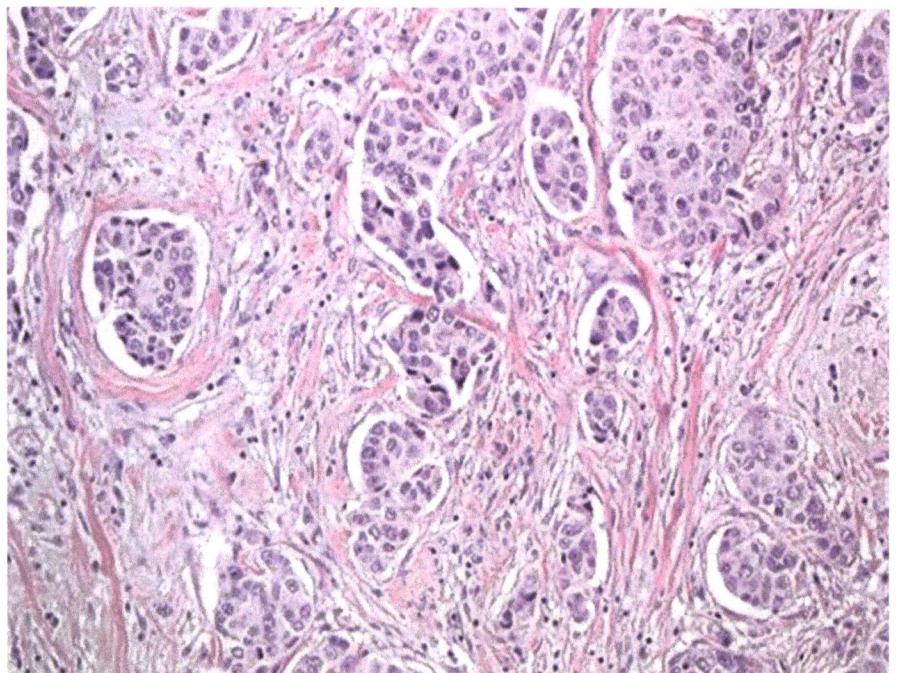

Fig. 10.27: Pathology result was ductal adenocarcinoma: Tumor cells in cords, solid or trabecular patterns.

CONCLUSION

Elastographic findings in concordance with pathology result.

Chapter 10: Interpretation of Malignant Breast Lesions 113

CASE 4: A 68-year-old woman referred for a palpable mass of the left breast.

Digital mammography findings have been shown in Figure 10.28.

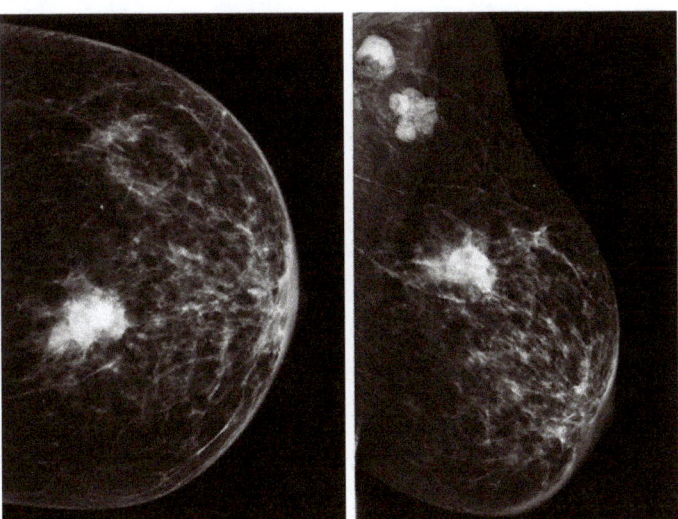

Fig. 10.28: MLO and CC view of left breast depicted an enlarged spiculated, irregular high-density mass, with skin thickening and associated unilateral, enlarged and dense, with loss of the hilum lymph nodes.

Physical examination: Palpable, painless, immobile mass 2.5 cm of the left breast.
B-mode ultrasound findings have been shown in Figure 10.29.

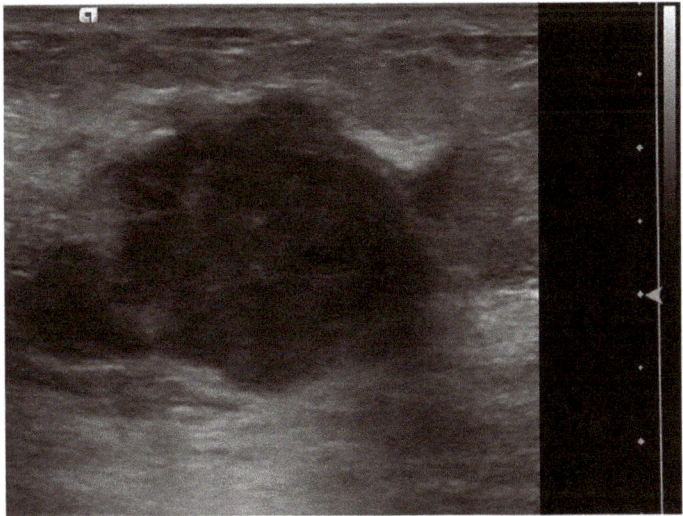

Fig. 10.29: B-mode ultrasound revealed a marked hypoechoic mass with indistinct margins and spiculations. There were also microcalcifications.

Color Doppler findings have been shown in Figure 10.30.

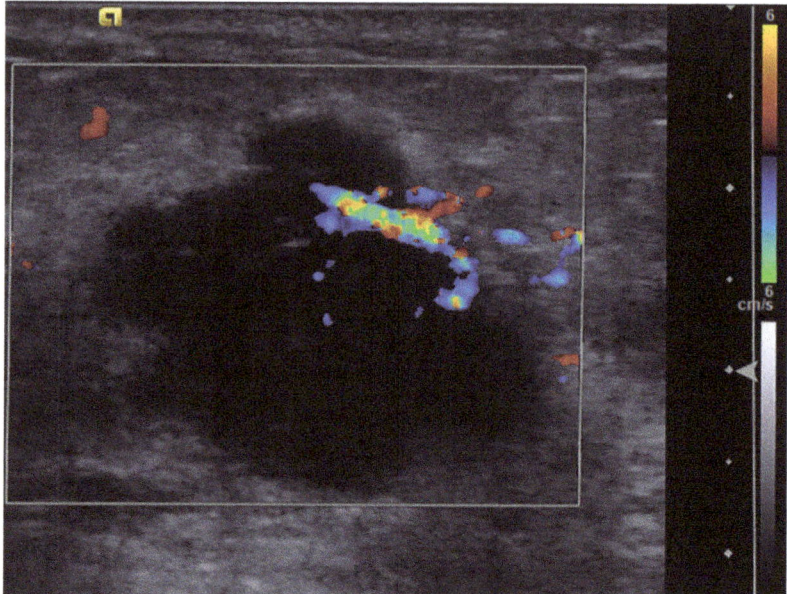

Fig. 10.30: Color Doppler depicted increased internal vascularity.

Grayscale strain imaging has been shown in Figure 10.31.

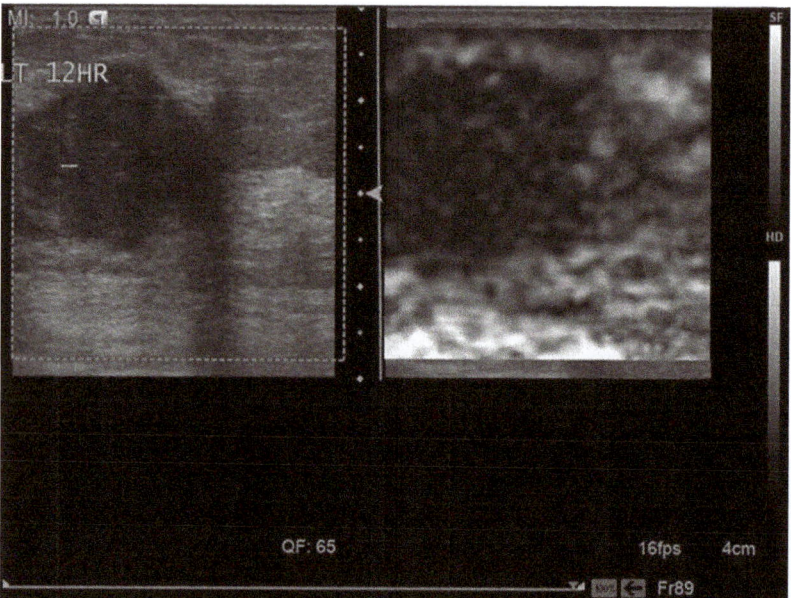

Fig. 10.31: The lesion appears stiffer than the surrounding tissue and also bigger than in B-mode (E/B >1).

Strain ratio estimation has been shown in Figure 10.32.

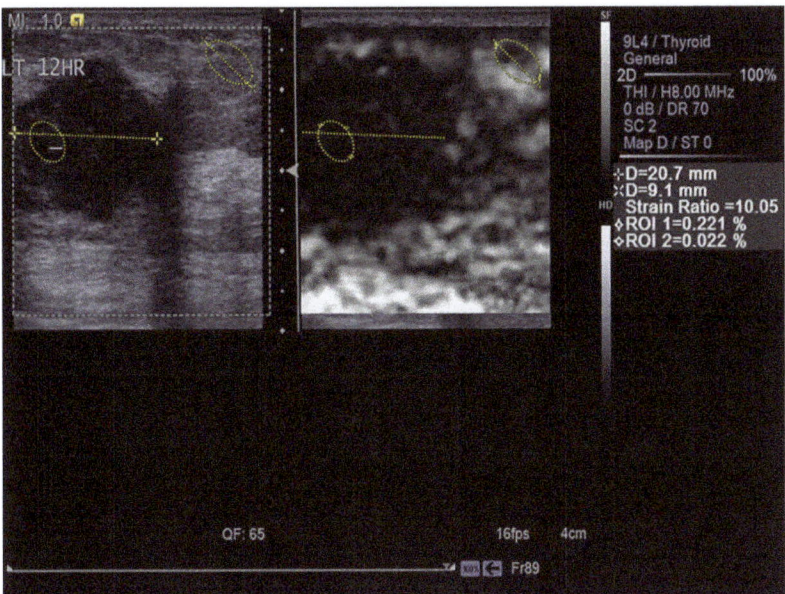

Fig. 10.32: Strain ratio is equal to 10.05.

Elasticity score has been shown in Figure 10.33.

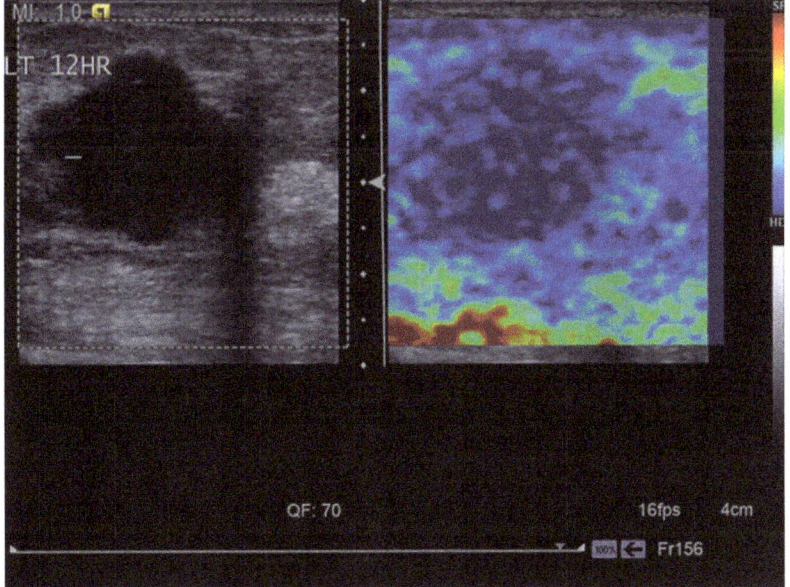

Fig. 10.33: Elasticity score is 5.

VTI grayscale imaging has been shown in Figure 10.34.

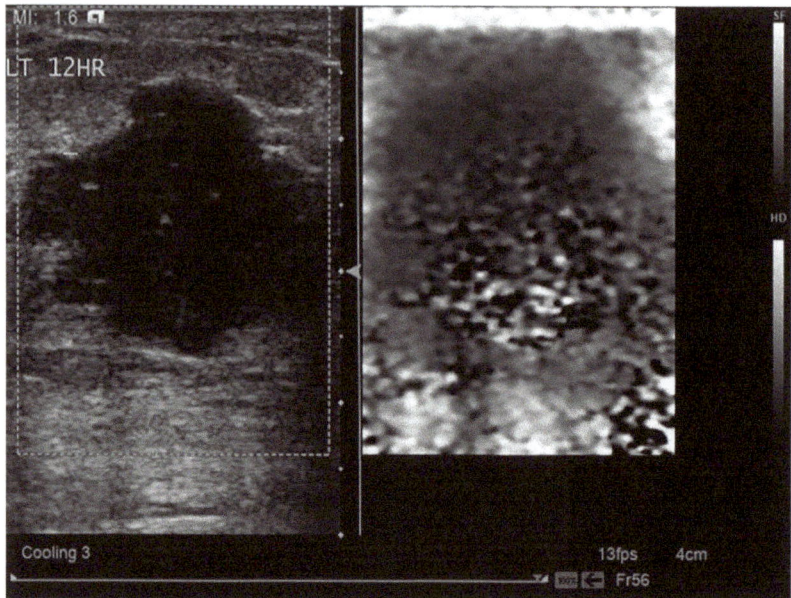

Fig. 10.34: The mass is depicted with the typical "cellular sample" image.

VTI color map imaging has been shown in Figure 10.35.

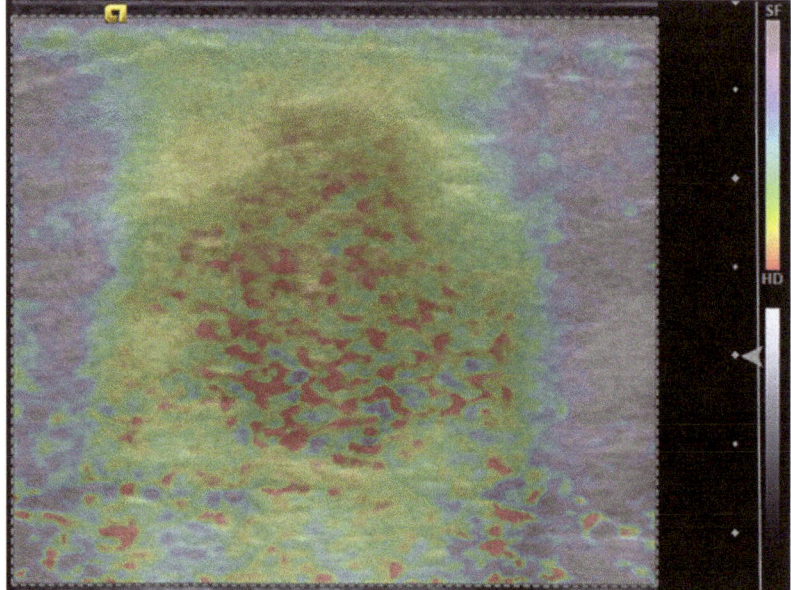

Fig. 10.35: The mass is depicted as red-green (= stiff).

VTQ value estimation inside the lesion has been shown in Figure 10.36.

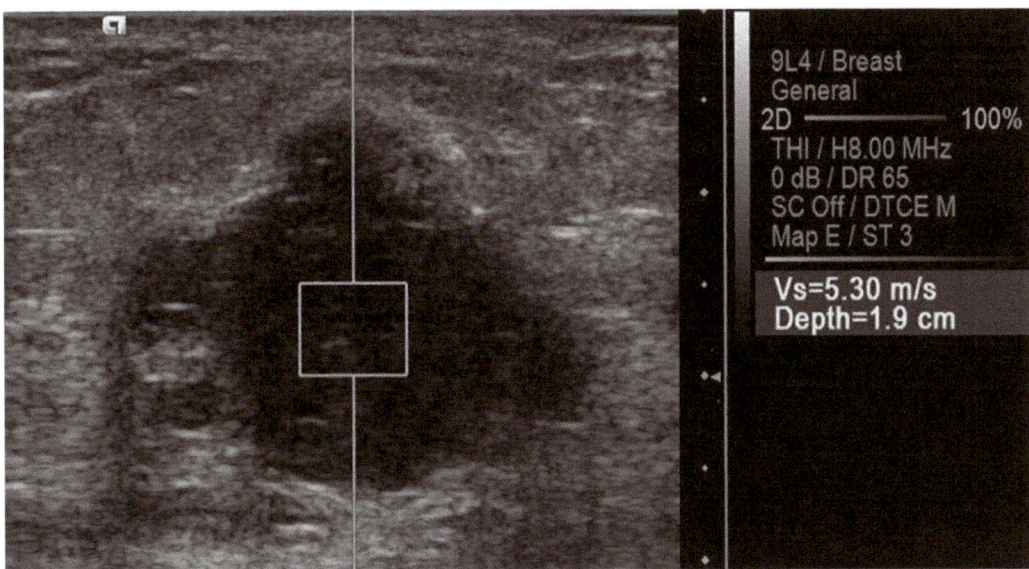

Fig. 10.36: Vs inside the lesion = 5.30 m/sec.

VTQ value estimation in the adjacent tissue has been shown in Figure 10.37.

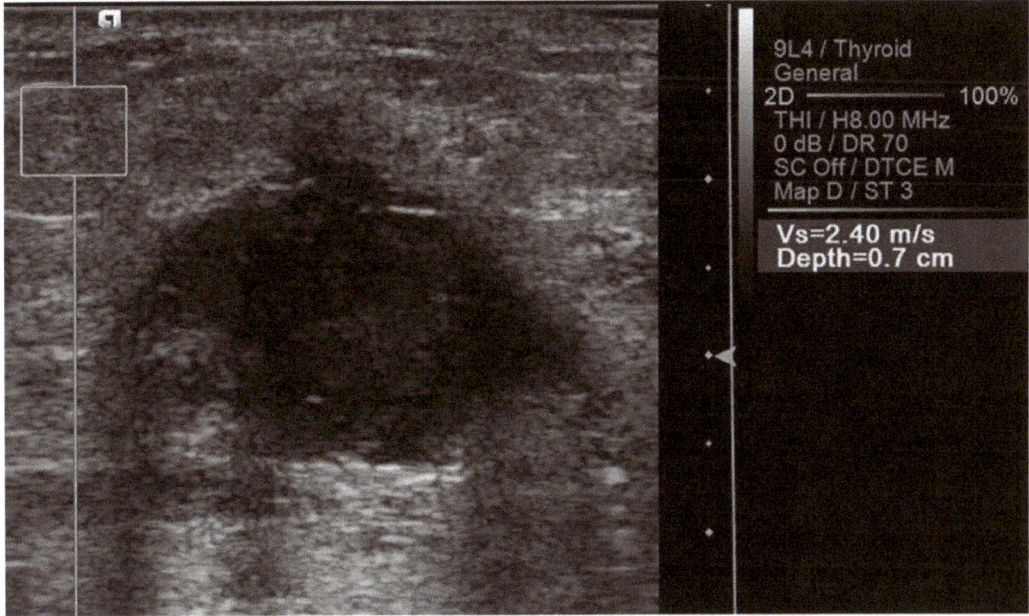

Fig. 10.37: Vs in the adjacent tissue = 2.40 m/sec.

Pathology result has been shown in Figure 10.38.

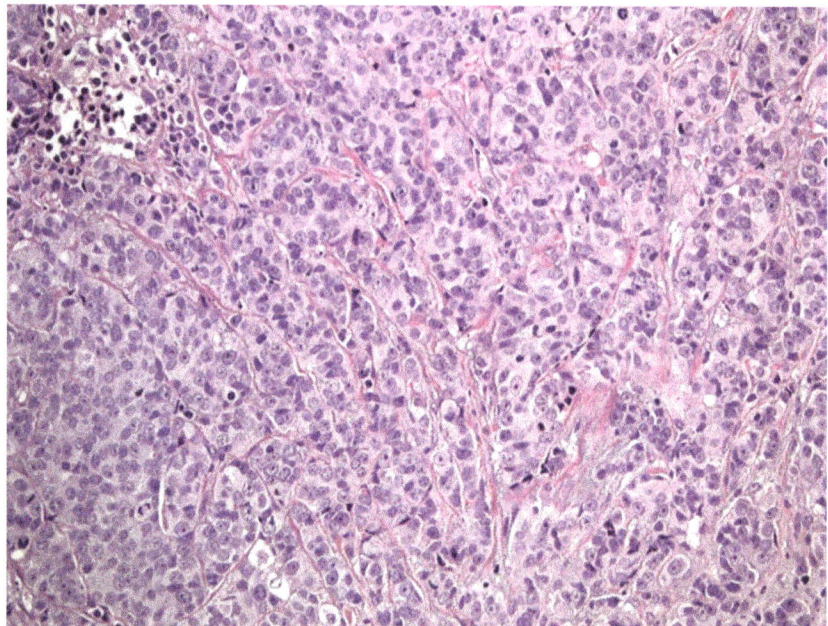

Fig. 10.38: Pathology result was ductal invasive carcinoma grade III.

CONCLUSION

Elastographic and pathology findings were in concordance.

CASE 5: A 56-year-old woman.

B-mode ultrasound findings have been shown in Figure 10.39.

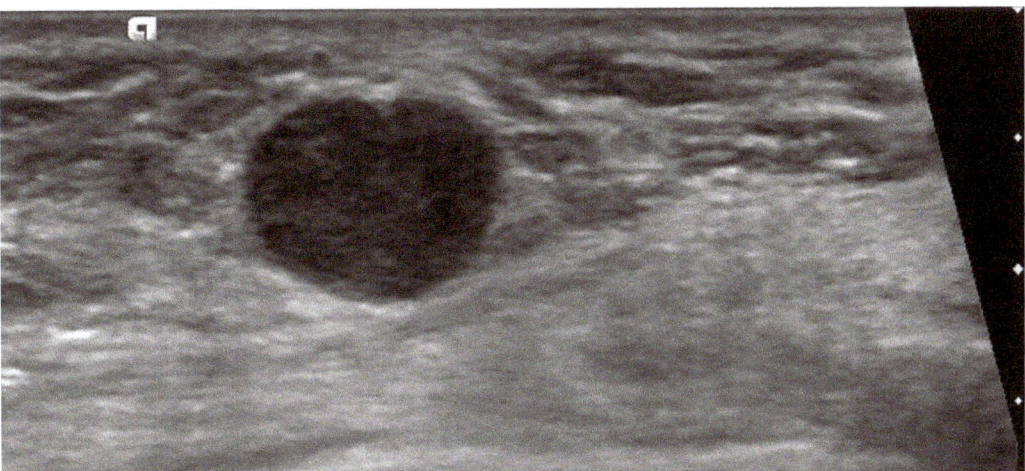

Fig. 10.39: B-mode revealed a round, hypoechoic, homogenous, and well-defined mass.

Color Doppler findings have been shown in Figure 10.40.

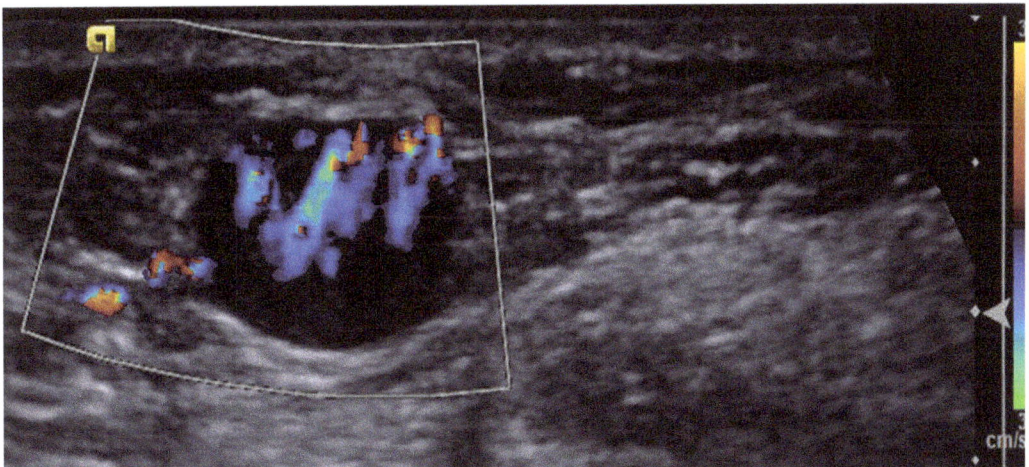

Fig. 10.40: The mass depicted with increased internal vascularity.

Grayscale strain imaging has been shown in Figure 10.41.

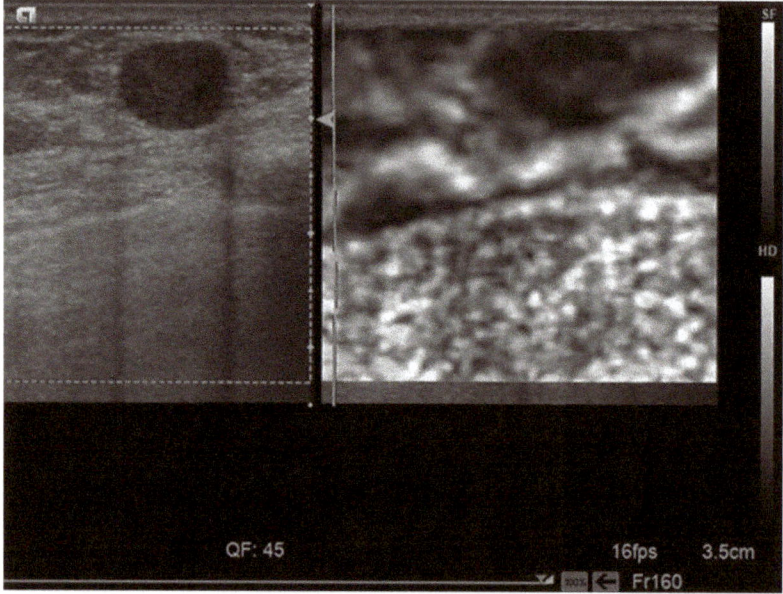

Fig. 10.41: The lesion appears stiffer than the surrounding tissue and bigger than in B-mode image.

Strain ratio calculation has been shown in Figure 10.42.

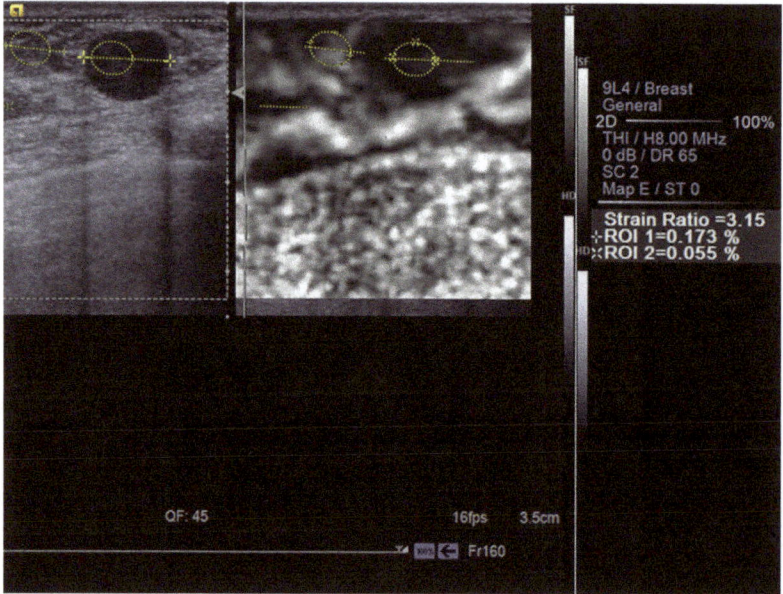

Fig. 10.42: Strain ratio is 3.15.

Elasticity score has been shown in Figure 10.43.

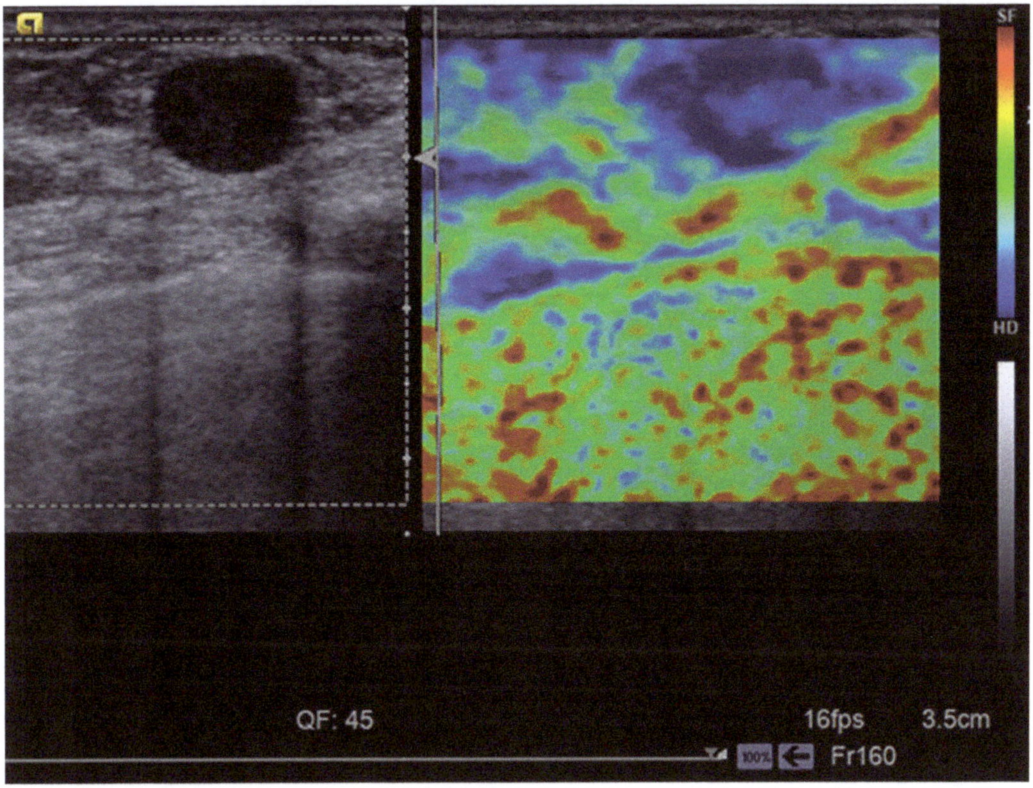

Fig. 10.43: Elasticity score is 4.

VTI grayscale imaging has been shown in Figure 10.44.

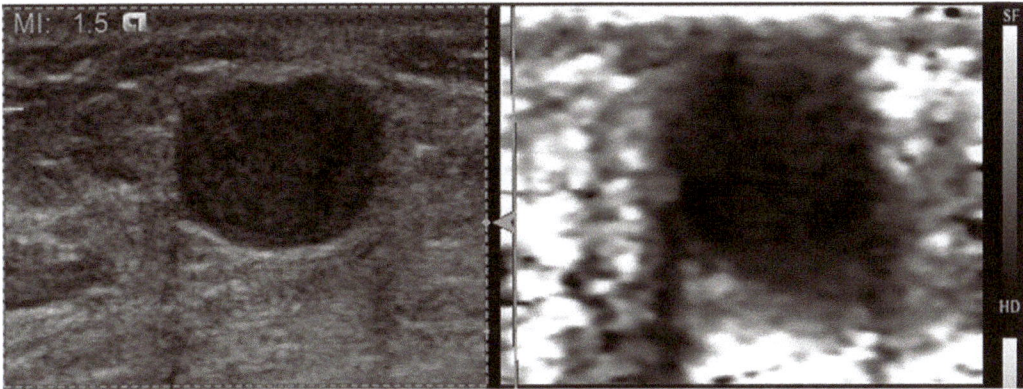

Fig. 10.44: The lesion is stiffer than the surrounding tissue.

VTI color map imaging has been shown in Figure 10.45.

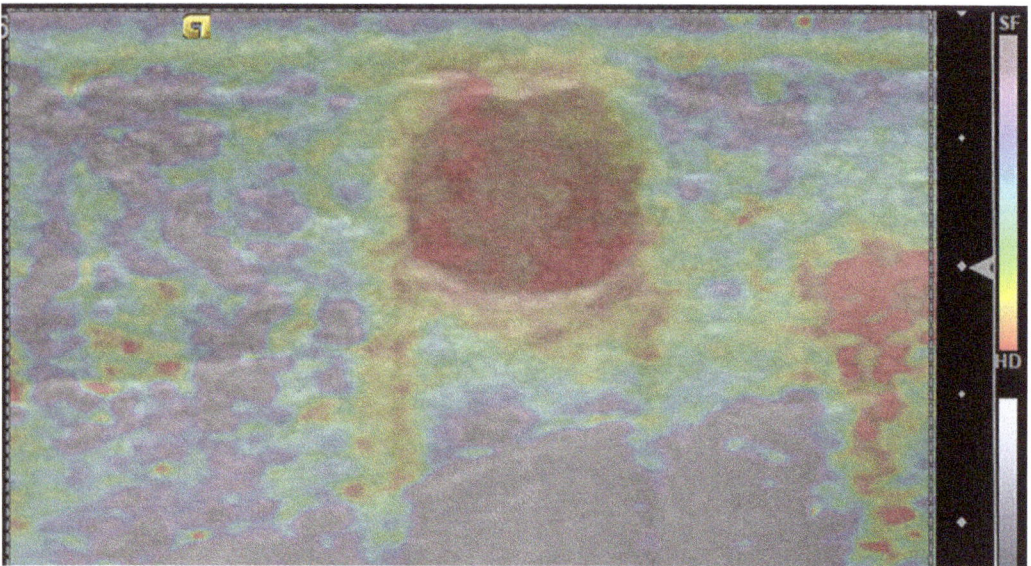

Fig. 10.45: The lesion appears red (= stiff).

VTQ value estimation inside the lesion has been shown in Figure 10.46.

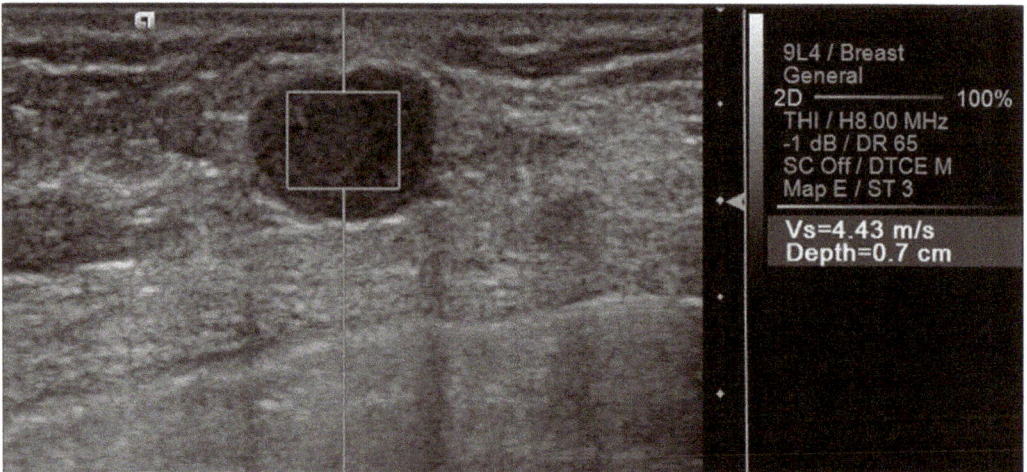

Fig. 10.46: Vs = 4.43 m/sec.

Chapter 10: Interpretation of Malignant Breast Lesions 123

VTQ value estimation in the adjacent tissue has been shown in Figure 10.47.

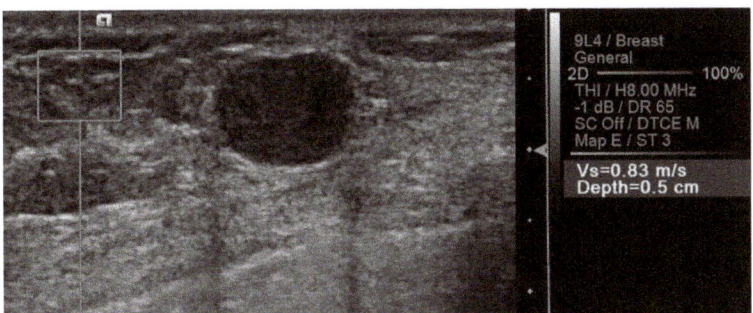

Fig. 10.47: Vs = 0.83 m/sec.

Pathology result has been shown in Figure 10.48.

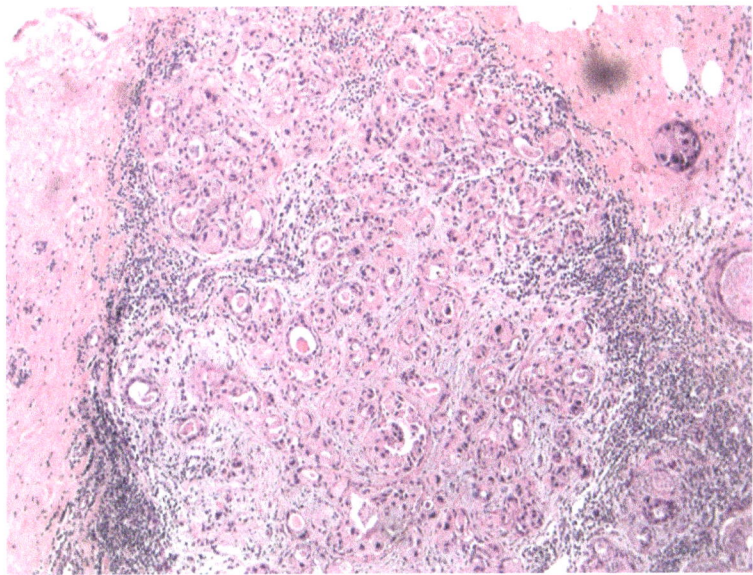

Fig. 10.48: Ductal adenocarcinoma with lobular cancerization.

CONCLUSION

B-mode ultrasound findings were suggestive of benignity. On the other hand, elastographic findings were suggestive of malignancy and in concordance with pathology result.

CASE 6: A 76-year-old woman referred for screening mammography.

Digital mammography findings have been shown in Figure 10.49.

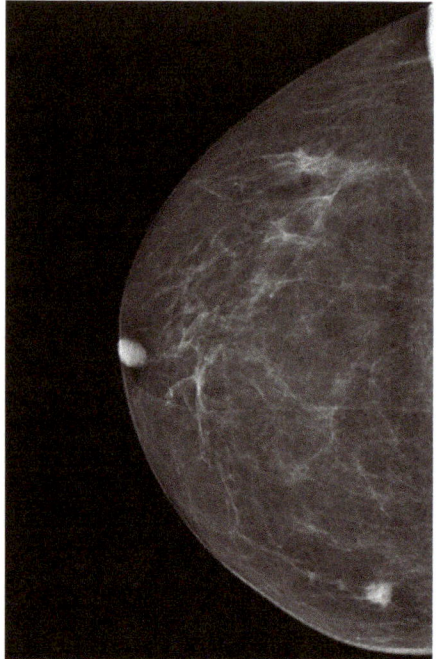

Fig. 10.49: CC view of right breast depicts a spiculated, irregular high-density mass.

B-mode ultrasound findings have been shown in Figure 10.50.

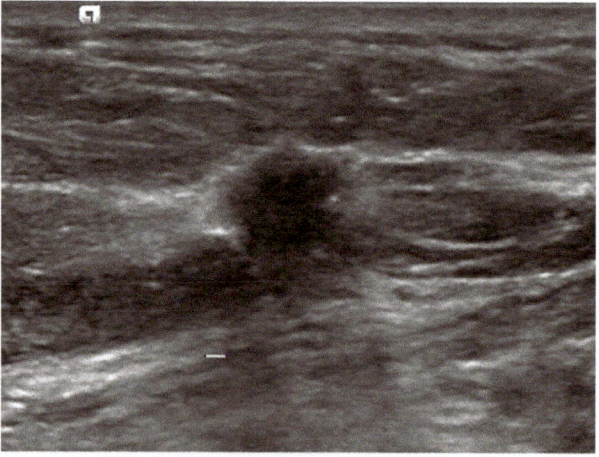

Fig. 10.50: B-mode US revealed a hypoechoic mass with irregular margins.

Grayscale strain imaging has been shown in Figure 10.51.

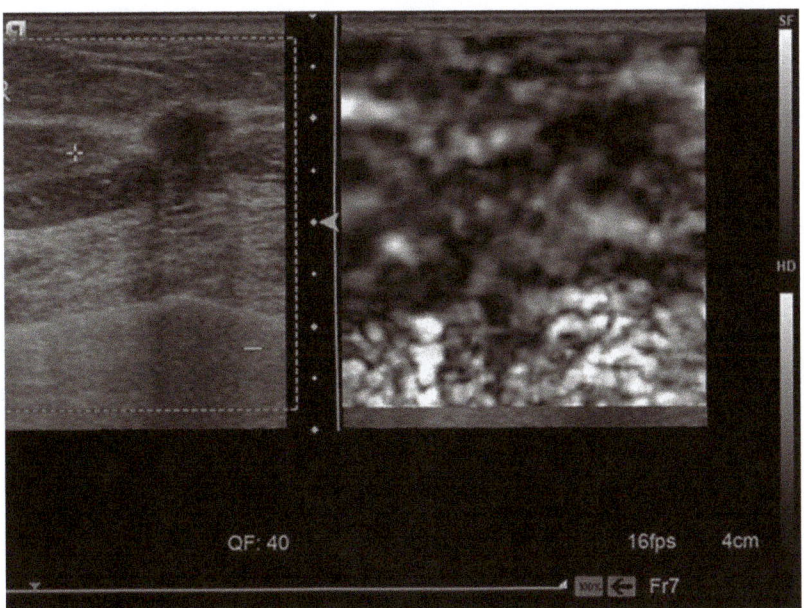

Fig. 10.51: The lesion is stiff with E/B greater than 1.

Strain ratio calculation has been shown in Figure 10.52.

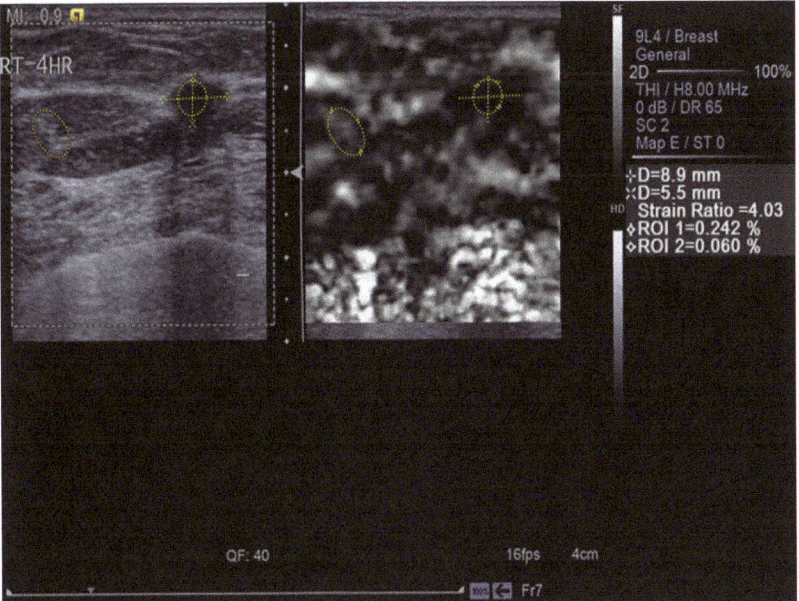

Fig. 10.52: Strain ratio is 4.03.

Elasticity score has been shown in Figure 10.53.

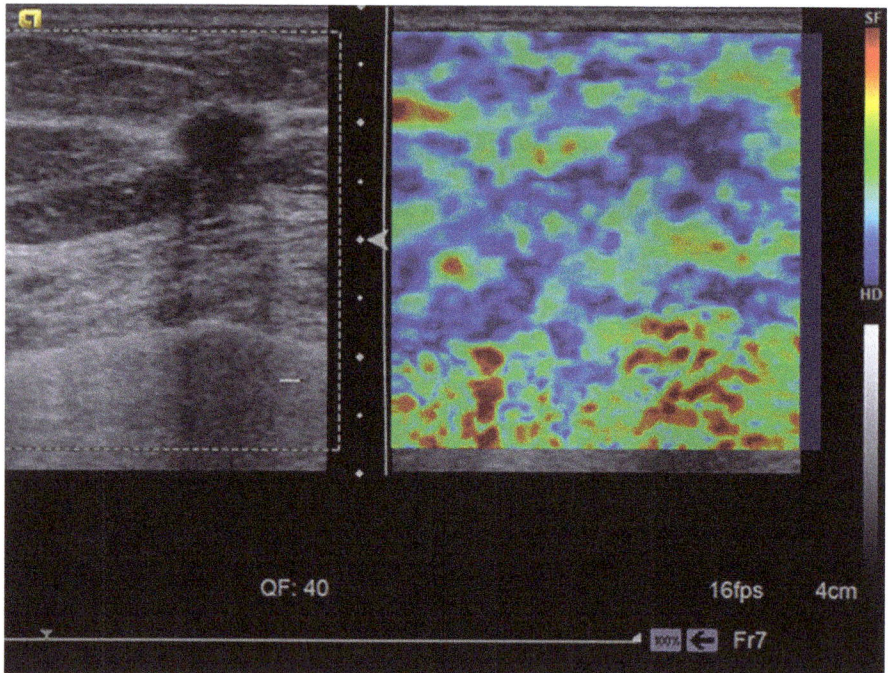

Fig. 10.53: Elasticity score is 4.

Grayscale VTI imaging has been shown in Figure 10.54.

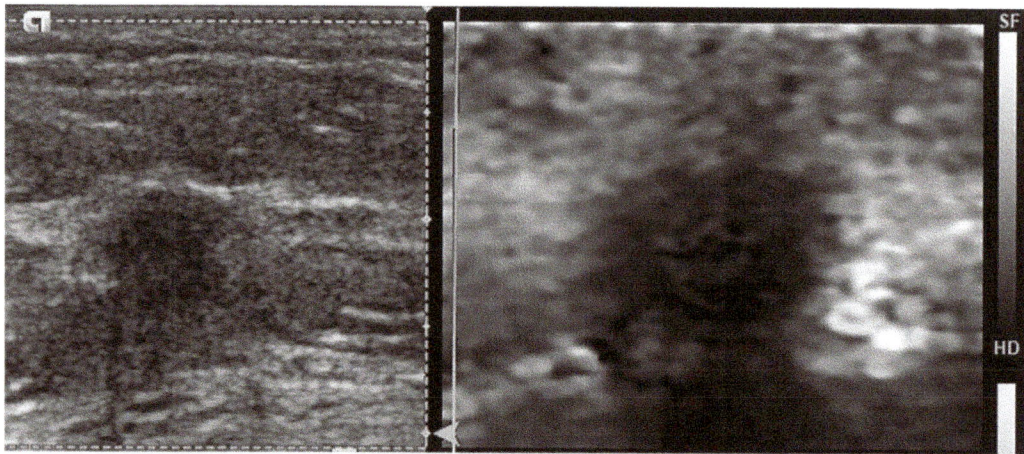

Fig. 10.54: The lesion appears stiffer than the surrounding tissue.

Color map VTI imaging has been shown in Figure 10.55.

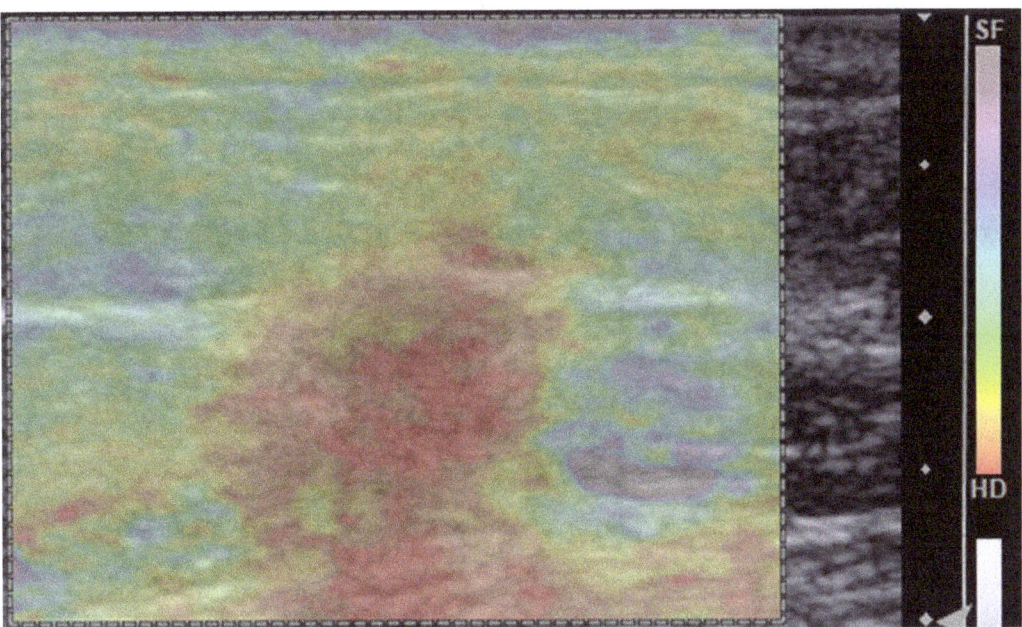

Fig. 10.55: The lesion is red (= stiff).

VTQ value estimation inside the lesion has been shown in Figure 10.56.

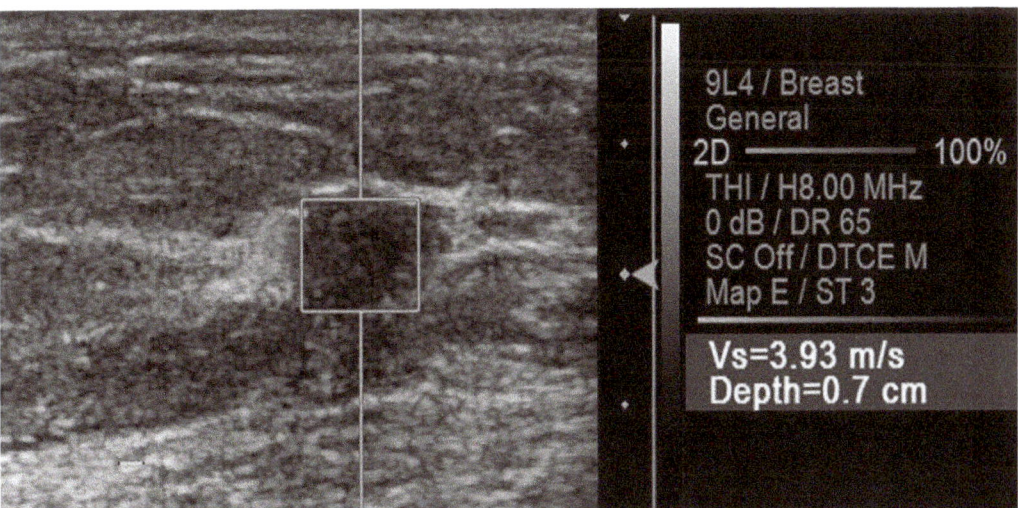

Fig. 10.56: Vs = 3.93 m/sec.

VTQ value estimation in the adjacent tissue has been shown in Figure 10.57.

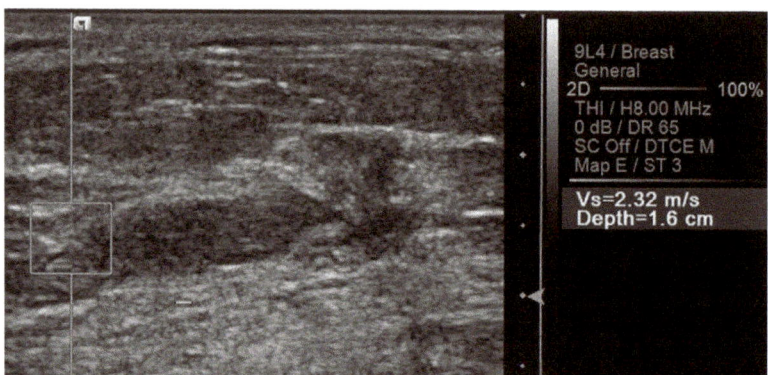

Fig. 10.57: Vs = 2.32 m/sec.

Pathology result has been shown in Figure 10.58.

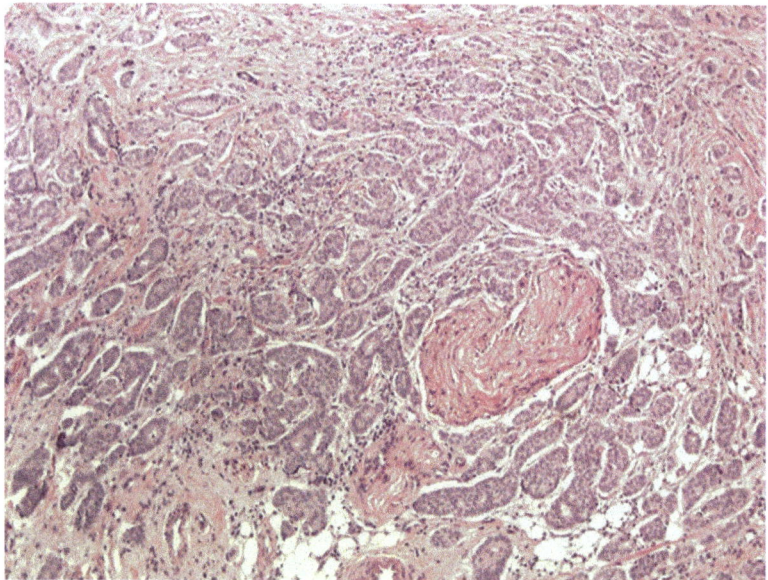

Fig. 10.58: Pathology result was invasive carcinoma NST grade II with perineural invasion (according to modified Nottingham grading system).

■ CONCLUSION

Elastographic and pathology results were in concordance.

In this case, it is important to keep in mind that because of the small size of the lesion the region of interest (ROI) must be inside the lesion and the surrounding tissue should not be included.

Chapter 10: Interpretation of Malignant Breast Lesions 129

CASE 7: A 64-year-old woman.

B-mode ultrasound findings have been shown in Figure 10.59.

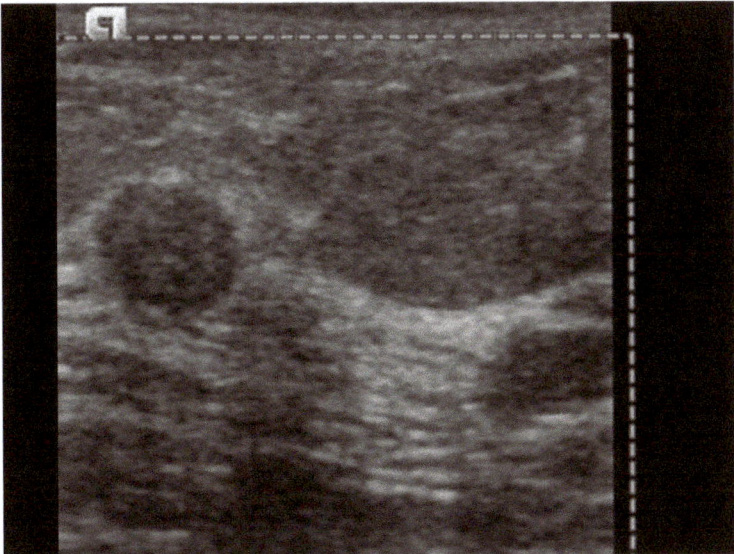

Fig. 10.59: Ultrasound revealed a round, slightly hypoechoic, well-circumscribed mass.

Strain ratio calculation has been shown in Figure 10.60.

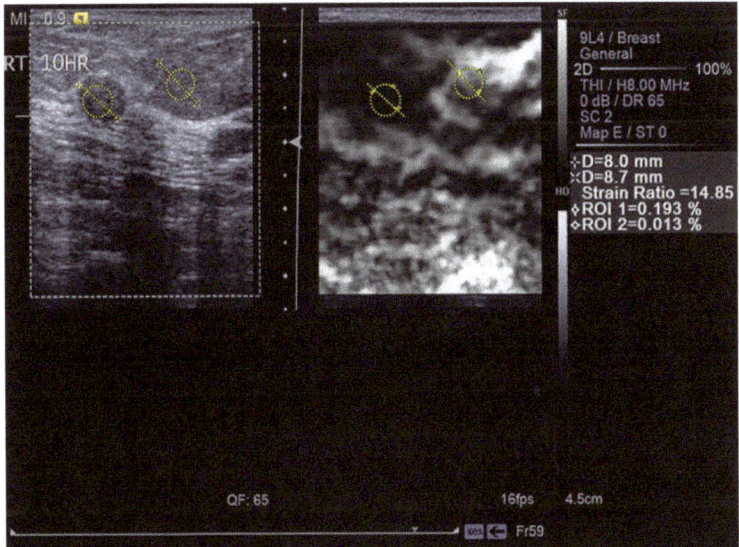

Fig. 10.60: Strain ratio is 14.85 (very high).

Elasticity score has been shown in Figure 10.61.

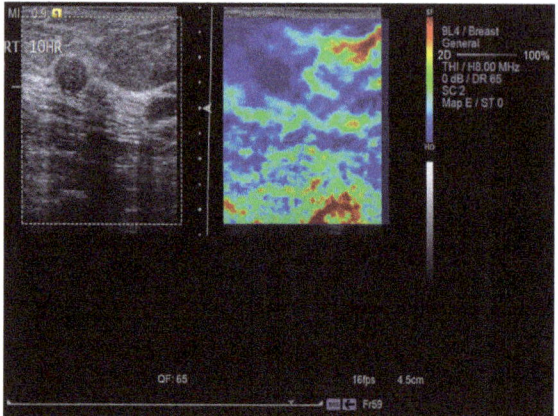

Fig. 10.61: Elasticity score is 5.

Grayscale VTI imaging has been shown in Figure 10.62.

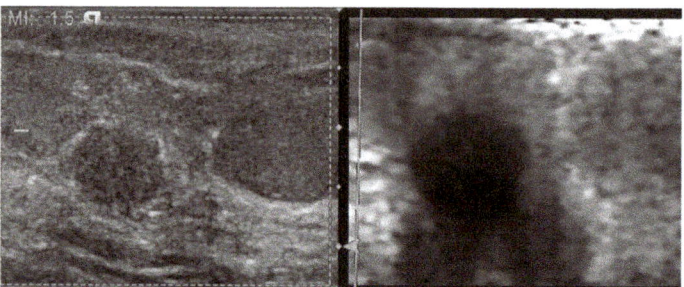

Fig. 10.62: The lesion is darker than the surrounding tissue.

Color map VTI imaging has been shown in Figure 10.63.

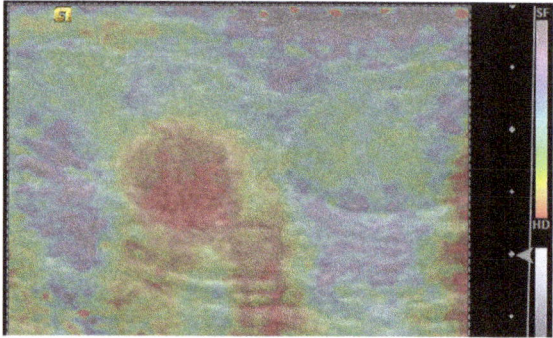

Fig. 10.63: The lesion is totally red.

Pathology result has been shown in Figure 10.64.

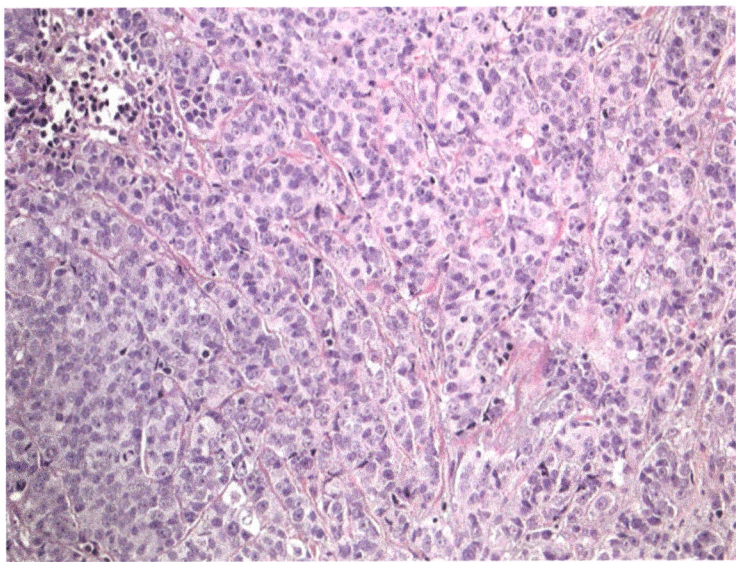

Fig. 10.64: Ductal invasive carcinoma grade III.

CONCLUSION

Although B-mode ultrasound findings were suggestive of a benign lesion, elastographic findings were indicative of malignancy and in concordance with pathology result.

SUGGESTED READING

Cutler SJ, Young JL (Eds). Third National Cancer Survey: Incidence Data. NCI monograph no. 41. Bethesda, Md: National Cancer Institute. 1975. pp. 413-4.

Giardini R, Piccolo C, Rilke F. Primary non-Hodgkin's lymphomas of the female breast. Cancer. 1992;69:725-35.

Gkali CA, Chalazonitis AN, Feida E, et al. Primary non-Hodgkin lymphoma of the breast: ultrasonography, elastography, digital mammography, contrast-enhanced digital mammography, and pathology findings. Ultrasound Q. 2015;31(4):279-82.

Schouten JT, Weese JL, Carbone PP. Lymphoma of the breast. Ann Surg. 1981;194:749-53.

CHAPTER 11 | Pitfalls

Christina An. Gkali

CASE 1: A 40-year-old woman referred for a palpable, painless mass of right breast.

B-mode ultrasound findings have been shown in Figure 11.1.

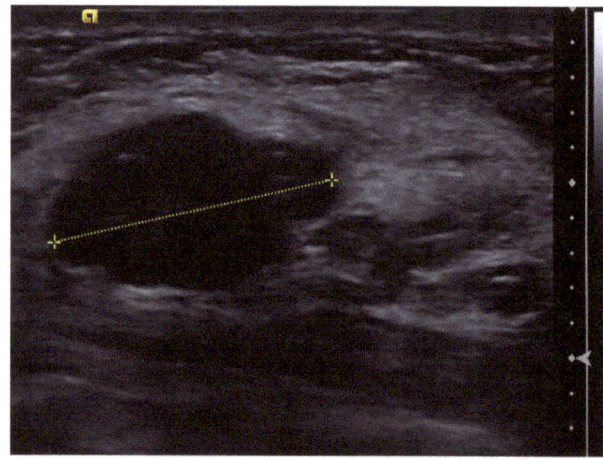

Fig. 11.1: B-mode ultrasound (US) revealed a hypoechoic, lobulated, well-circumscribed mass, measured 1.7 cm in maximum diameter. Macrocalcifications were present.

Virtual touch quantification (VTQ) value estimation inside the lesion has been shown in Figure 11.2.

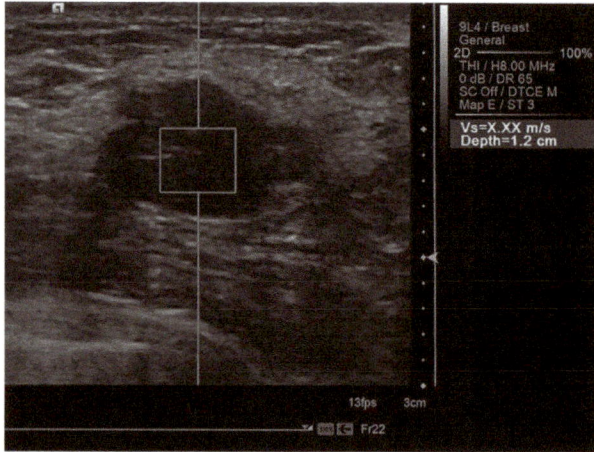

Fig. 11.2: Vs inside the lesion was demonstrated as X.XX m/sec.

The reason for the inability to calculate the Vs inside the lesion is due to the presence of macrocalcifications.

Note: Vs inside the lesion were demonstrated as x.xx m/sec.

When a lesion contains calcifications that are visible, the region of interest (ROI) should be placed out of them, if it is possible, so the Vs inside the lesion can be estimated.

Pathology result has been shown in Figure 11.3.

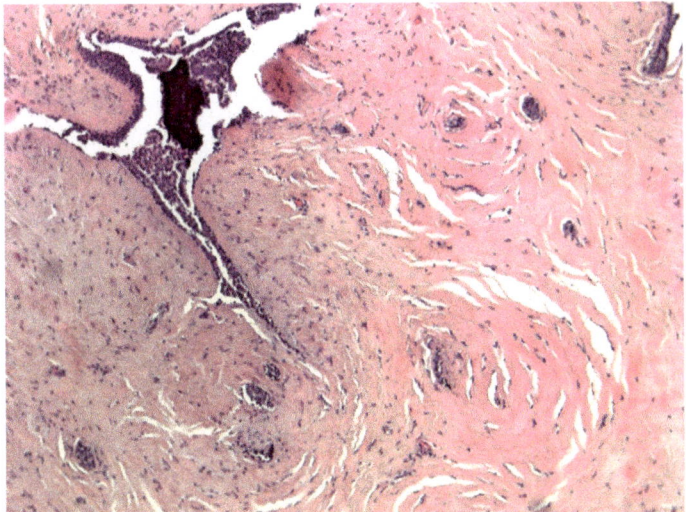

Fig. 11.3: Pathology result was fibroadenoma with calcification surrounded by epithelium.

CASE 2: A 20-year-old girl referred for evaluation of a palpable, painful mass of her right breast.

Physical examination: Palpable mass, approximately 2 cm with associated localized breast edema, erythema, warmth, and pain.

B-mode ultrasound findings have been shown in Figure 11.4.

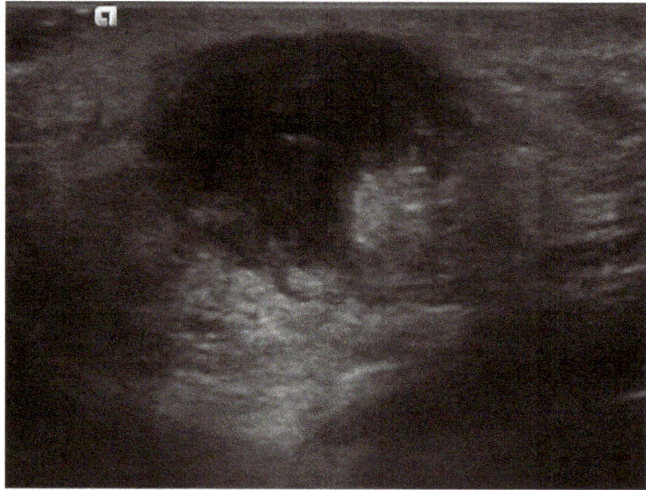

Fig. 11.4: B-mode ultrasound revealed a 2 cm in maximum diameter, mixed mass (anechoic with internal echoes), with irregular margins, posterior enhancement and no internal septae.

Virtual touch quantification value estimation inside the lesion has been shown in Figure 11.5.

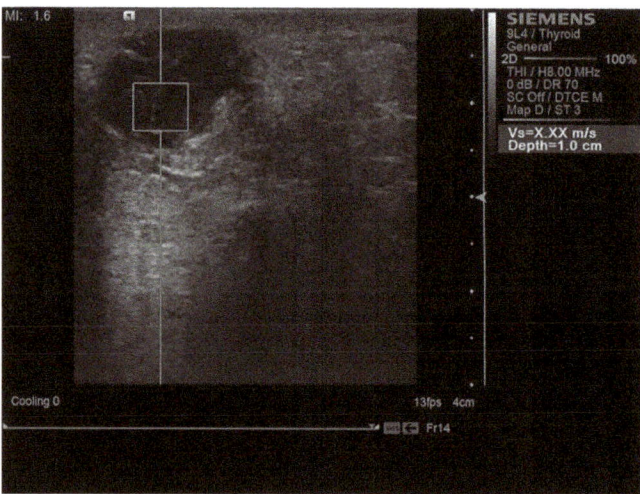

Fig. 11.5: VTQ value was impossible to be calculated and was displayed as X.XX m/sec.

Pathology result has been shown in Figure 11.6.

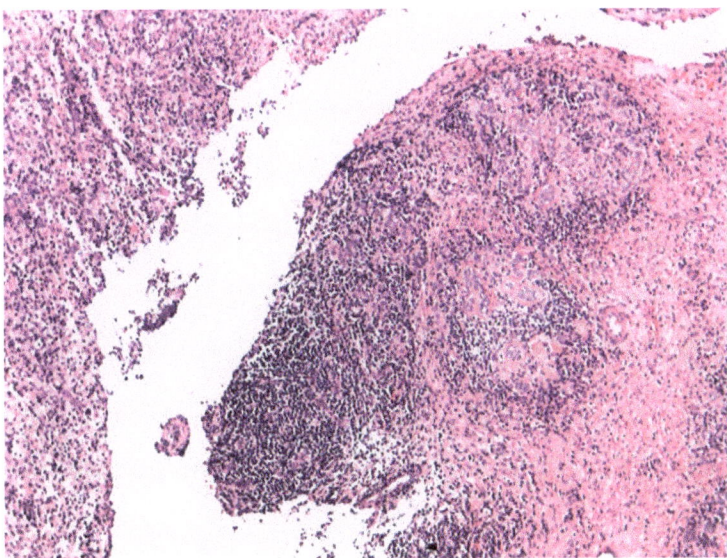

Fig. 11.6: Breast tissue is displaced by chronic active inflammation with lymphocytes, plasma cells, and neutrophils.

Abscesses because of their heterogeneity in their composition may result in a signal that is not accurately identified and this is why VTQ value inside the lesion was impossible to be evaluated and demonstrated as X.XX m/sec.

CASE 3: A 75-year-old woman.

B-mode ultrasound findings have been shown in Figure 11.7.

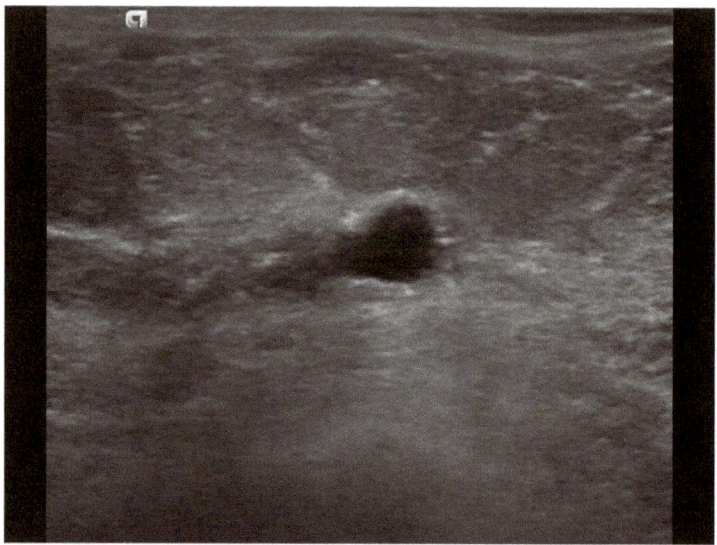

Fig. 11.7: B-mode ultrasound revealed a hypoechoic lesion with indistinct margins.

Strain ratio calculation has been shown in Figure 11.8.

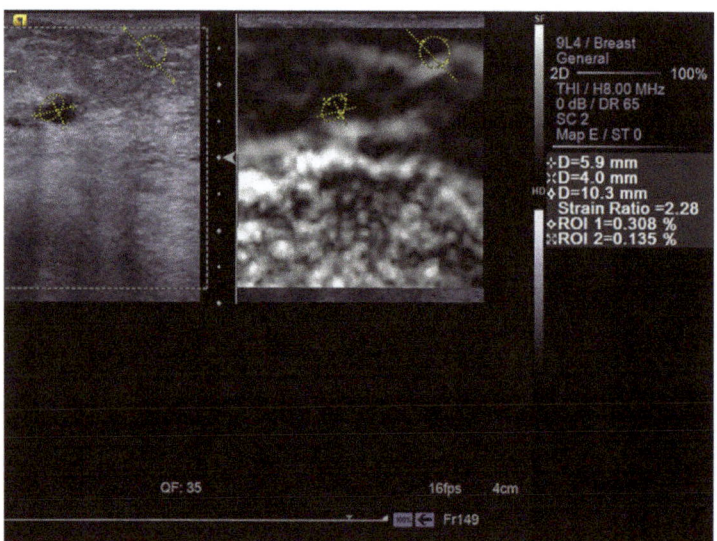

Fig. 11.8: Strain ratio was equal to 2.28. But you can notice that ROI of the lesion includes normal surrounding tissue because the lesion is too small.

Virtual touch quantification value estimation inside the lesion has been shown in Figure 11.9.

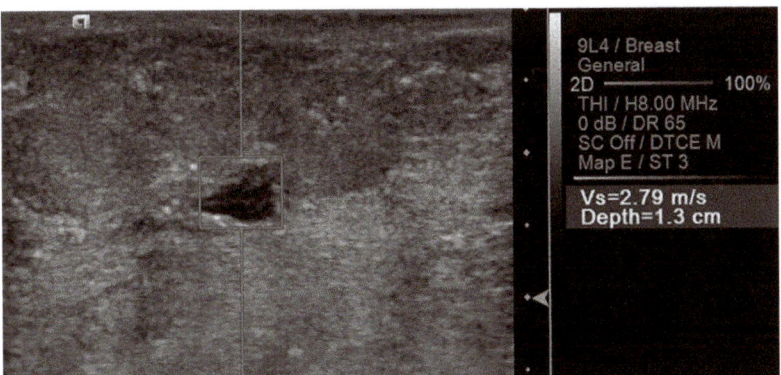

Fig. 11.9: Vs inside the lesion was estimated 2.79 m/sec.

Pathology result has been shown in Figure 11.10.

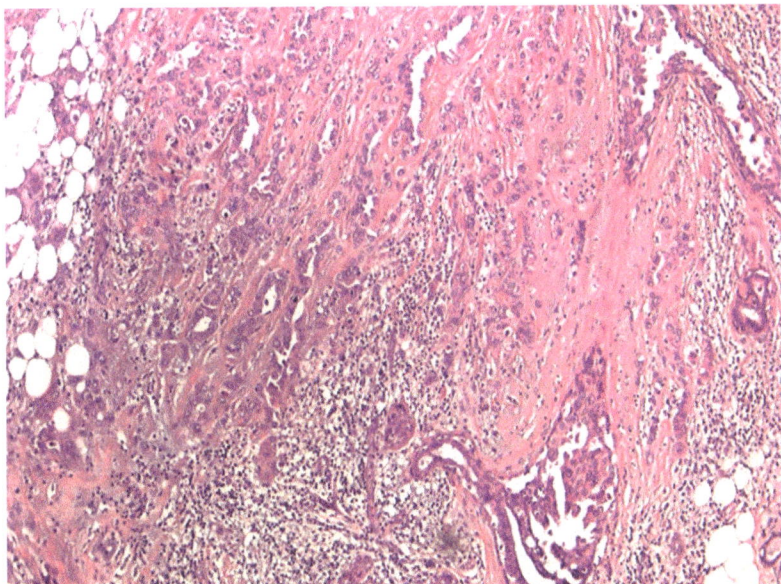

Fig. 11.10: Pathology result was coexistent invasive and intraepithelial ductal carcinoma.

The lesion was small enough to be included in the ROI and this resulted in wrong estimation of Vs inside the lesion. Although the lesion was malignant, the estimated Vs was low because normal surrounding tissue was included inside the ROI.

Although small ROI resulted in wrong estimation of both Vs inside the lesion and strain ratio elasticity score and virtual touch imaging (VTI) (both grayscale and color map) were suggestive of malignancy.

Elasticity score has been shown in Figure 11.11.

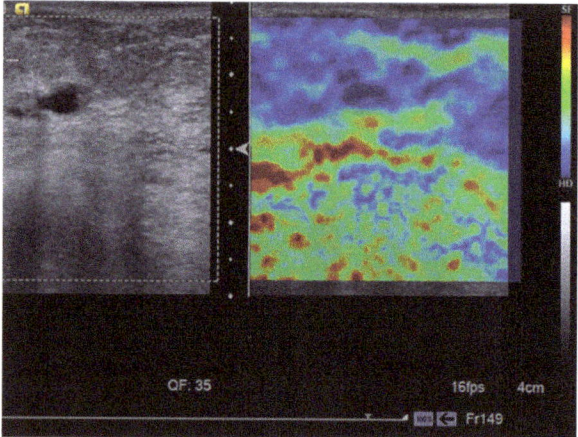

Fig. 11.11: Elasticity score is 4.

Grayscale VTI imaging has been shown in Figure 11.12.

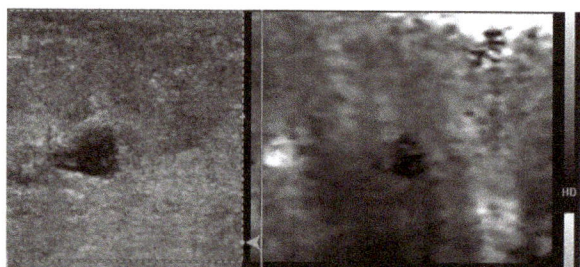

Fig. 11.12: The lesion is depicted darker than the surrounding tissue.

Color map VTI imaging has been shown in Figure 11.13.

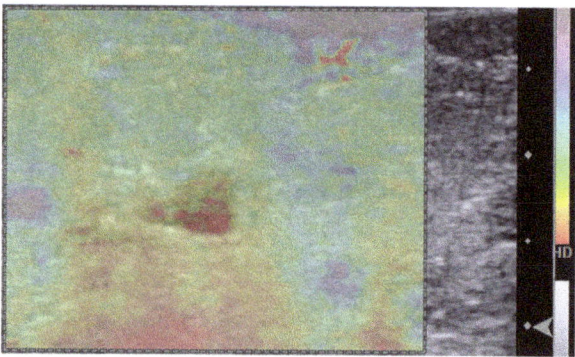

Fig. 11.13: The lesion is depicted red (= stiff).

Chapter 11: Pitfalls 139

CASE 4: A 71-year-old referred for a palpable mass.

B-mode ultrasound findings have been shown in Figure 11.14.

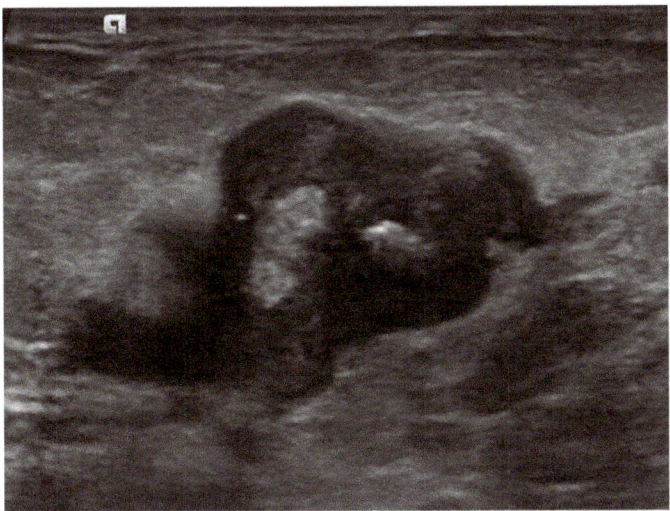

Fig. 11.14: Ultrasound revealed a hypoechoic, lobulated mass with indistinct margins and presence of microcalcifications.

Although elasticity score and VTI imaging (both grayscale and color map) were indicative of malignancy, Vs inside the lesion was impossible to be calculated because of the presence of macrocalcifications (Fig. 11.15).

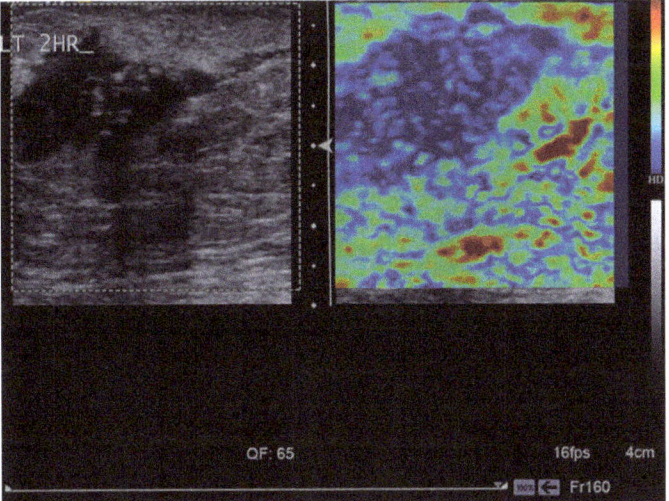

Fig. 11.15: Elasticity score is 1.

Grayscale VTI imaging has been shown in Figure 11.16.

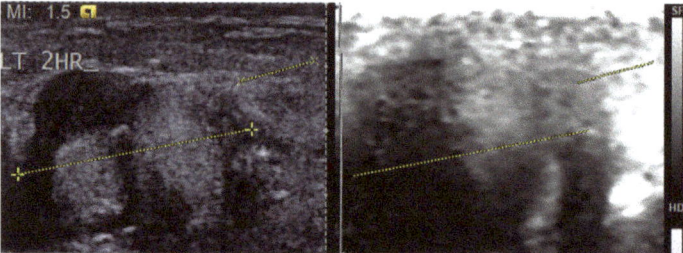

Fig. 11.16: The lesion is darker than the surrounding tissue.

Color map VTI imaging has been shown in Figure 11.17.

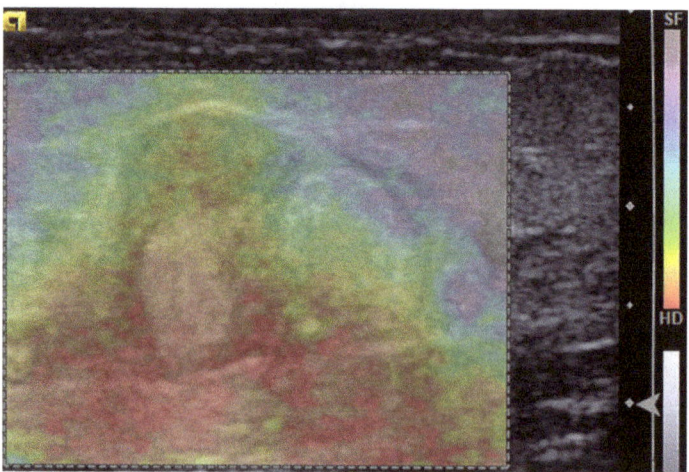

Fig. 11.17: The lesion is depicted red-yellow (= stiff).

Virtual touch quantification value estimation inside the lesion has been shown in Figure 11.18.

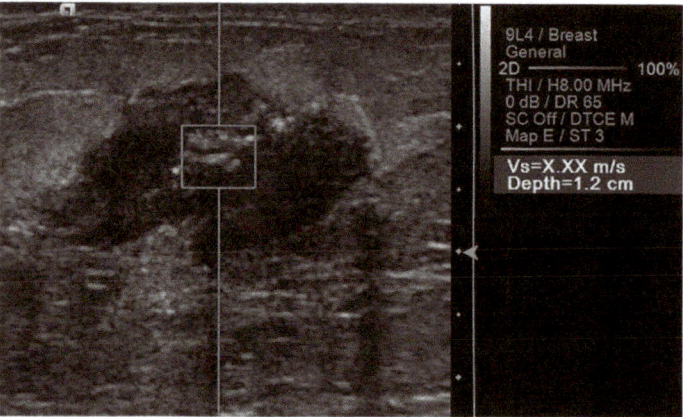

Fig. 11.18: Vs was impossible to be estimated because of the presence of macrocalcifications.

Index

Page numbers followed by f refer to figure

A

Acoustic push pulses 36f
  multiple 47f
Acoustic radiation force impulse 12, 15, 35, 49, 55, 56, 93
  beam 36f
  elastography 16f
Acquisition tips 30, 31, 50
Adenomyoepithelioma 84f
Adenosis 80f
Adipose cell 4
Alpha-smooth muscle actin 8
Alveolar epithelial cell 4
Androgen receptors 5
Anechoic with internal echoes 134f
Axillary lymph node 105f

B

B-cell origin 103f
  of breast 102f
Biopsy-proven
  fibroadenoma 24f, 26f, 27f
  myoepithelioma 27f
B-mode ultrasound 61, 63
Breast
  cancer 11
  classification on right 99f
  ductal system 3f
  imaging reporting and data system 8, 11, 25
  lactating 6f
  left 77f, 85, 94f, 113f
  lesions
    benign 59, 61
    malignant 59, 99
  painful mass of right 63, 89, 132, 134
  palpable mass of left 81, 94, 113
  pathological and surgical approach 1
  postmenopausal 7f
  postoperative image of 93f
  premenopausal 7f
  right 99, 104f, 124f
  tissue 38f, 45f, 66f, 135f
  ultrasound elastography reporting 53, 55
Bull's eye
  artifact 98f
  sign 25f

C

Capillary vessel 4
Cardiac pulsations 21f
Color Doppler 64
Cyst 25
  complicated 25f
Cytokeratins, low molecular weight 5

D

Deoxyribonucleic acid 8
Duct
  lobular unit, terminal 3, 4f, 5f
  segmental 3
Ductal adenocarcinoma 112f, 123f
  pathology-proven 45f, 46f
Ductal carcinoma in situ 6, 21
Ductal epithelial cell 4

E

Elasticity score 64, 68, 78, 96, 101, 106, 106f, 110, 110f, 115, 115f, 121, 126, 130, 138
Elastography 12, 15
  basic principles of 13
  compression 16f
  works 16
Encapsulated mass 67f
Epithelium 133f
Estrogen receptor-alpha 5, 7

F

Fatty hilum, loss of normal 105f
Fibroadenoma 71f, 88f
    pathology-proven 37f, 38f, 42f, 43f, 46f
Fibroblast 4
    activated protein 8
Fibrofatty breast tissue 102f
Fine-needle aspiration cytology 92
Florid adenosis 88f

G

Grayscale strain 22f
    elastography 62
    imaging 105, 114, 120, 125
Grayscale virtual touch imaging 69, 74, 83, 87, 90, 110, 126, 130, 138, 140

H

Hilum lymph nodes, loss of 113f
Human epidermal growth factor receptor 7
Hypercellular mesenchymal component 98f
Hypocellular stroma 71f
Hypoechoic mass 13f, 23f, 27f, 40f, 41f, 100f, 104f, 109f

I

Ill-defined mass 28f
Immune cell 4
Inflammation
    chronic active 135f
    with lymphocytes 66f
Intraepithelial ductal carcinoma 108f, 137f
Invasive ductal carcinoma, pathology-proven 39f, 42f

J

Juvenile fibroadenoma 93f

L

Lactiferous sinus 3
Lobular hyperplasia 6f
Lymph node 108f
    cortex 105f
Lymphocytes 135f
Lymphoma cells 102f

M

Molecular weight cytokeratins, high 5
Muscle myosin heavy chain, smooth 5
Myoepithelial cell 4, 5f
    layers 84f

N

Neutrophils 66f, 135f
Non-Hodgkin's lymphoma 102f

P

Phosphoinositide 3-kinase 8
Phyllodes tumor 98f
Pitfalls 132
Plasma cells 66f, 135f

R

Region of interest 16, 24, 30, 31, 35, 49, 50, 74, 128, 133
    grayscale imaging 116, 121
Respiration 21f

S

Screening digital mammography 67
Shear strain 17f
Signal-to-noise ratio 48
Strain 18f
Strain elastography 30
    imaging 30
Strain imaging 19, 21, 55

Strain ratio 24, 30, 106f, 115f
    calculation 95, 106, 109, 120, 125, 129, 136
    estimation 115
    evaluation 65
Stress 18f
Subsegmental duct 3

T

Tissue strain 15, 21f
    physics of 16
Tubular adenoma, pathology-proven 38f
Tumor cells 103f
    in cords 112f

V

Virtual touch
    image in grayscale 35
    imaging 37, 35, 107, 137
    quantification 12, 43, 49, 50, 65, 70, 71, 91, 102, 132, 134, 137, 140
        value estimation 75, 79, 84, 87, 88, 97, 108, 111, 117, 122, 123, 127
    tissue
        imaging 12, 49, 55, 56
        quantification value 56

www.ingramcontent.com/pod-product-compliance
Lightning Source LLC
Chambersburg PA
CBHW040541220526
45473CB00016B/2993